THE NUTRiBASE COMPLETE

FAST FOOD RESTAURANT

NUTRITION COUNTER

THE NutriBase COMPLETE

FAST FOOD RESTAURANT

NUTRITION COUNTER

DR. ART ULENE

Avery Publishing Group

Garden City Park, New York

The information in this book is based upon the latest data made available by government agencies, food manufacturers, and trade associations. It is important to note that all nutrient breakdowns for processed foods are subject to change by manufacturers without notice and may therefore vary from printing to printing.

ISBN 0-89529-666-7

Printed in the United States of America

10   9   8   7   6   5   4   3

CONTENTS

INTRODUCTION

During the last few years, we have begun to understand the many ways in which the foods we eat can affect the quality of our health and the length of our life. This new health- and food-consciousness has spurred the publication of numerous books and articles that clearly explain how we can plan meals and cook foods to maximize nutrition and health. Most of these publications, of course, focus on meals prepared at home. Although generally not stated, it is usually assumed that meals eaten in restaurants—and, most especially, in fast food restaurants—are too high in fat, and often too low in nutrients, to have a place in a healthful diet.

Because of today's busy lifestyles, though, fast food restaurants are often the "dining rooms" of choice for many Americans. And in response to the country's growing interest in health, many of these restaurants have enlarged their offerings by adding green salads, skinless chicken parts, leaner burgers, and a variety of other healthier dishes to their menus. By being aware of the many options available and making wise choices, it is now possible to limit fat and calories, and maximize fiber and other nutrients—even when eating breakfast, lunch, or dinner on the run!

This book was designed to help you do just that. It enables you to learn more about the foods you should consume—or avoid—so you can choose those foods that will contribute to your good health.

When using this book, don't be intimidated by the huge number of choices listed or by the impossible-to-memorize nutritional value numbers that accompany the lists. It is not necessary to memorize these numbers. Instead, just try to familiarize yourself with the restaurant foods that are best suited to your needs. Begin by looking up the foods you eat most often. If these foods are not providing you with the nutrients you're looking for, use the book to find better alternatives that are just as tasty. You'll be surprised by how easy it is to learn about these foods and to make any necessary changes.

As you take more control over the foods you are eating and put more thought into your choices, keep in mind that good nutrition is just one element of a healthy lifestyle. To achieve maximum health, your life should be filled with physical activity and free of cigarette smoke and other toxic substances. In addition, the stress in your life should be under control. Even the best diet can't overcome the problems caused by smoking, an immoderate use of alcohol, poorly managed stress, and other health-compromising habits.

Finally, keep in mind that research is constantly adding to our knowledge of nutrition, and, in the process, changing some of our beliefs. As best you can, try to keep up with the new information and, when appropriate, make whatever dietary changes are necessary. But also be skeptical about nutritional news that seems too good to be true. (More often than not, it isn't true.) Be wary of nutritional claims made by people who are trying to sell you something. And be cautious—don't make any drastic changes in your nutritional program without first talking to a health professional who is knowledgeable about nutrition and about your particular medical circumstances. Don't forget: If the right nutritional choices are powerful enough to keep you well, it is only logical that the wrong ones could make you sick.

The following section will explain some of the basics of nutrition. After that, you will learn how to use this book to locate the information you need to improve your diet.

A QUICK LOOK AT SOME IMPORTANT NUTRIENTS

Everyone's diet must contain certain basic nutrients, including carbohydrates, proteins, and fats. In addition, recent research has indicated that other food components—such as fiber and cholesterol—are important in their own ways. A proper balance of these essentials is necessary for optimum health.

This book presents selected nutrient values of a wide range of restaurant foods. In order to wisely use this information, it is helpful to have a basic understanding of the function of the nutrients included in the book.

Carbohydrates

Carbohydrates are divided into two groups—simple carbohydrates and complex carbohydrates. *Simple carbohydrates,* sometimes called simple sugars, are found in large amounts in fruits. *Complex carbohydrates,* which include fiber and starches, are plentiful in vegetables, whole grains, peas, and beans.

Except for fiber, which is a type of carbohydrate that cannot be digested, both simple and complex carbohydrates are converted into glucose, which is either used directly to provide energy for the body, or stored in the body for future use. Thus, carbohydrates are the main source of blood glucose, which is a major fuel for all of our cells, and the only source of energy for the brain and red blood cells.

Fiber

As mentioned earlier, fiber is actually a type of carbohydrate. Yet the importance of fiber is so great that it merits special attention.

Dietary fiber—referred to in the past as "roughage"—is found in foods that come from plants, especially vegetables, fruits, whole grain breads and cereals, brown rice, and beans and legumes. Although fiber is actually the part of plant materials that our body cannot digest, this substance is known to perform a number of important functions. It promotes feelings of fullness; prevents constipation, hemorrhoids, and other intestinal problems; and is associated with a reduced incidence of colon cancer. In addition, high-fiber diets help lower blood cholesterol levels, thereby reducing the risk of heart disease. (To learn about the difference between crude fiber and dietary fiber, see page xv.)

Protein

Protein is essential for growth and development. It provides the body with energy, and is needed for the manufacture of hormones, antibodies, enzymes, and muscle tissues. It also helps maintain the proper acid-alkali balance in the body. Inadequate protein intake can result in stunted growth, diarrhea, vomiting, lack of appetite, and edema, a buildup of fluids in the tissues.

The foods richest in protein include milk, eggs, cheese, fish, meat, and poultry. Other good sources are whole grains, nuts, beans, and peas.

Fat and Cholesterol

Recently, much attention has been focused on the need to reduce dietary fat. Nevertheless, the body does need fats—but only the right fats, and only in appropriate quantities. Specifically, it needs fatty acids, which perform a variety of vital bodily functions. Fatty acids carry the fat-soluble vitamins. They are essential for growth and development, and for the maintenance of healthy skin, hair, and nails. And they provide the body with energy. A variety of problems occur when the body fails to receive adequate fatty acids. Signs of this deficiency may include retarded growth; skin, hair, and nail disorders; and an impaired metabolism of fats and fat-soluble vitamins.

Although fat is necessary, most of us are now aware that there are several kinds of dietary fat—saturated, polyunsaturated, and monounsaturated—and that some are better than others. To understand the difference between these three fats, it is helpful to first learn a little about cholesterol.

Cholesterol is a white, waxy, fatty substance found in all foods that come from animal sources. Cholesterol is essential to our well-being, as it helps to build cell membranes, to produce hormones, and to manufacture bile acids. The liver is capable of manufacturing all of the cholesterol needed for good health.

The cholesterol manufactured by our liver is carried through our bloodstream by LDLs (low-density lipoproteins). High levels of LDLs in the bloodstream can result in clogged arteries, causing high blood pressure, stroke, or heart disease. This is why LDL is referred to as the "bad" cholesterol. Fortunately, in many people, LDL levels can be reduced to healthy levels through proper diet.

HDLs (high-density lipoproteins) carry excess cholesterol from different body tissues to the liver, where it is converted to bile acids and then eliminated through the intestines. High levels of HDLs are linked with a decreased risk of coronary heart disease. This is why HDL is often called the "good" cholesterol. To a limited extent, HDL levels can be raised through regular exercise.

How are the three types of fat related to cholesterol? Saturated fats—which come from animal foods like meat, fish, poultry, milk, butter, and cheese, as well as from palm, coconut, and palm kernel oil—have been shown to increase total blood cholesterol levels, especially the undesirable LDL portion. Polyunsaturated fats—found mainly in vegetable oils like corn, sunflower, safflower, and soybean—tend to lower levels of both HDLs and LDLs. Monounsaturated fats—found mainly in vegetable and nut oils such as olive, peanut, and canola—have been shown to reduce total blood cholesterol without lowering levels of the good cholesterol, HDL. Indeed, some monounsaturated fats have been shown to raise HDL levels.

One other element, trans-fatty acids, might also play a role in blood cholesterol levels. Trans-fatty acids occur when polyunsaturated oils are altered through hydrogenation, a process used to harden liquid vegetable oils into solid foods like margarine and shortening. One recent study found that trans-monounsaturated fatty acids raise LDL cholesterol levels, behaving much like saturated fats. Simultaneously, these trans-fatty acids reduce HDL cholesterol readings. Much more research is necessary, since some studies have not produced clear-cut conclusions about these substances. For now, however, it is clear that when your goal is to lower cholesterol, polyunsaturated and monounsaturated fats are much more desirable than saturated fats. In fact, there is no biological need for saturated fat!

Sodium

Sodium helps maintain normal fluid levels in the body, is involved in healthy muscle functioning, and supports the blood and lymph systems. Fainting, intolerance to heat, headaches, muscle cramps, and swelling in the extremities may all result from an inadequate intake of sodium.

It is important to note, though, that most people get too *much* sodium in their diet. Because an excessive intake of sodium can cause hypertension (high blood pressure), and can aggravate many medical disorders, including congestive heart failure, certain forms of kidney disease, and premenstrual syndrome (PMS), nutritionists recommend a maximum intake of about 2,400 milligrams of sodium per day.

Calories

When we talk about foods, we often mention the number of calories a certain food has. Calories, though, are not a nutrient, like fat or protein. What, then, are they?

A calorie is an energy unit. As already discussed, carbohydrates, protein, and fat provide the body with the energy it needs to function. This energy is measured in calories. There are, for instance, 4 calories in every gram of protein, 4 calories in every gram of carbohydrate, and 9 calories in every gram of fat. It is no wonder, then, that when people try to lose weight, they are often advised to cut down on fatty foods. On a gram-for-gram basis, fat is more than twice as fattening as carbohydrates or protein.

In addition to fat's having more calories than protein or carbohydrates, it is important to understand that the way in which our body metabolizes dietary fat is different from the way it metabolizes the other two nutrients. Because dietary fat is similar in chemical composition to body fat, it takes less energy to convert it to body fat. In fact, it takes only 3 percent of the calories in the fat we eat to turn that food into body fat, while it takes at least 25 percent of the carbohydrates and protein calories we eat to convert them into body fat. Remember, though, that if you eat more calories than your body needs, regardless of the nutrient providing these calories, the excess will be stored as body fat.

THE FOOD GUIDE PYRAMID

Over the years, the United States Department of Agriculture (USDA) has tried to ensure adequate nutrition by encouraging Americans to eat a "well-balanced diet"—a concept that has changed dramatically over the years. Most of us still remember the four food groups that the USDA once promoted. These food groups—fruits and vegetables; breads and cereals; meat, poultry, fish, and eggs; and dairy products—were developed to encourage a balanced diet that was rich in meat, poultry, and dairy products. Clearly, we now have a greater understanding of how such a diet affects our health, and the government now recommends a diet high in complex carbohydrates and low in fat. With this in mind, in May 1992, the government abandoned the four food groups in favor of

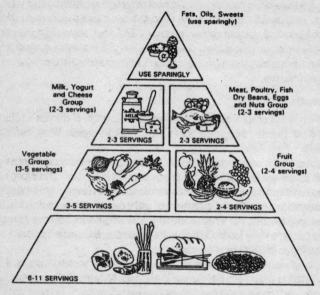

The Food Guide Pyramid

the Food Guide Pyramid, which has dramatically changed the recommended amounts of foods in each group.

At the base of the Food Guide Pyramid is the bread, cereal, rice, and pasta group. Six to eleven servings from this group are recommended daily—more servings than from any other food group. The next level of the pyramid is occupied by the vegetable group, with three to five daily servings recommended daily, and the fruit group, with two to four servings recommended daily. Moving upward, the next pyramid level is shared by the milk, yogurt, and cheese group—two to three servings—and the meat, poultry, fish, dry beans, eggs, and nuts group—two to three servings. Finally, at the peak of the pyramid are fats, oils, and sweets, a group of foods which is to be eaten only sparingly.

Scaling the Pyramid

To ensure that you have adequate servings of healthful foods, it is best to follow the Food Guide Pyramid and, within each group, to choose foods that are high in the nutrients needed for good health. The remainder of this book shows how each restaurant item rates in terms of total calories, protein content, carbohydrate content, and several other important components. The following guidelines will further help you to choose foods that meet your dietary needs. Included also are tips for ordering in fast food restaurants.

■ When eating foods from the important bread, cereal, rice, and pasta group, try to choose whole-grain, high-fiber, low-fat breads and cereals—preferably without added sugar, coloring, or unnecessary preservatives. Choose brown rice over white rice, and whole-wheat or other whole-grain pastas over pastas made from white flour.

■ When eating fruits and vegetables, eat fresh raw produce as often as possible. Water-soluble vitamins, such as vitamin C, may leach out of foods during cooking, be damaged by overprocessing, or be destroyed when foods are overcooked. Even fat-soluble vitamins, which are fairly stable during low-temperature cooking, can be affected by frying. When available, choose vegetables that have been steamed or microwaved rather than boiled or fried.

■ When choosing foods from the milk, yogurt, and cheese group, select low-fat and nonfat brands, which provide the most nutrients and the least amount of fat. When eating meat, poultry, and fish, choose the leanest cuts available, and select baked and broiled dishes rather than fried foods.

■ Select as few foods as possible from the fats, oils, and sweets group. When you do use fats and oils, though, choose monounsaturated and polyunsaturated fats instead of saturated fats. Limit your intake of sweets, often choosing fresh fruits instead of cakes, cookies, and other high-fat desserts.

■ Review restaurant offerings, and go only to those restaurants that provide foods whose nutrients will meet your dietary needs. For instance, you might want to choose a restaurant that offers a variety of fresh salads rather than one which serves mostly high-fat meat dishes.

■ Become familiar with the different options offered in any one restaurant. The same piece of chicken you order fried might be just as delicious—and substantially lower in calories and fat—when roasted.

■ Instead of ordering the special burger *and* the fried onion rings, order one or the other—the one you simply can't live without—and accompany it with a green salad or a baked potato. This will limit the fat in your meal, and help ensure adequate nutrients.

■ Eat slowly. Especially when eating in fast food restaurants, it's common to rush through a meal. If you take your time, though, you're likely to be more satisfied by less food.

The following section should provide you with the details you need to better access and understand the data contained in this volume. I hope that this book will inspire you to learn more about your unique nutritional needs and the foods you are using to meet those needs. You will enjoy the sense of control this knowledge gives you. More important, you will make better food choices and take a major step toward better health. Best wishes for good health always.

Arthur Ulene, MD

HOW TO USE THIS BOOK

This book was designed to provide comprehensive nutritional information on a wide range of national and regional restaurant chain foods. Because scientific techniques are constantly being improved and nutritional theory continues to advance, this book will be continuously updated to reflect the most current nutritional data available.

FINDING THE LISTING YOU WANT

This easy-to-use guide is an A-to-Z reference to the nutrient values of restaurant chain foods. Foods are listed alphabetically under the name of the appropriate restaurant, and each food item is accompanied by the amount of calories, protein, carbohydrates, sodium, fiber, fat, saturated fat, and cholesterol, as well as the percentage of calories that come from fat.

After you locate the listing of the food you are interested in, you may find that abbreviations have been used to provide you with the information you need. Refer to page xix for a complete key to the abbreviations used throughout this book.

UNDERSTANDING FIBER VALUES

When looking at the fiber values of foods, it is important to understand that as a result of two different methods of analysis, two different types of fiber have been listed in this book. For many years, the acid-based process used to measure the fiber content of foods actually destroyed some of the fiber it was designed to measure. Referred to as "crude fiber," the results of this type of analysis are inaccurate, and almost always show an amount that is lower than the actual amount of fiber present in the food. Later, a more precise enzyme-related process for measuring this nutrient was devised. The fiber analyzed with this system is referred to as "dietary fiber."

In the interest of accuracy, whenever possible, we have provided the most up-to-date, accurate measure of total dietary fiber. You will know that the value reflects *total fiber* when the number is not accompanied by a qualifying symbol. Unfortunately, in the case of a few foods, only the *crude fiber* value is available at this time. You will know that the value reflects crude fiber when it is preceded by the symbol >—meaning "greater than"—and followed by the letter c—meaning "crude." Of course, as techniques of analysis are improved and as additional foods are tested, the listings in this book will be updated.

UNDERSTANDING FAT PERCENTAGES

One feature that sets this book apart from many other nutrition books is the inclusion of the column called " % Calories From Fat." Although scientists and nutritionists can use any of several methods to determine this value, the simplest and most popular one is the "4-4-9 method." This technique assumes that 1 gram of protein contains 4 calories, that 1 gram of carbohydrate contains 4 calories, and that 1 gram of fat contains 9 calories. In beverages or other foods containing alcohol, it is assumed that each gram of alcohol contains 7 calories. Once you know the total calories and the calories from fat, the calculations used to determine the percentage of calories from fat is, in theory, fairly straightforward and accurate.

When applied to actual published nutrition data, however, several factors make the 4-4-9 method less than ideal. For one thing, many manufacturers consider any nutrient containing fewer than 5 calories to be "nutritionally insignificant." For this reason, the manufacturers "round off" their published values for protein, carbohydrates, and fats. Sometimes they publish a value of "<1.0 gram" of fat, which means that the fat content might be anywhere from 0.0 grams to 0.99 grams. When a food item contains only a few calories, the "insignificant" rounding of fat values can have significant and misleading consequences.

A consequence of this practice of rounding off values is that when the calorie values for protein, carbohydrates, and fat are added up, they very rarely match the calorie values published by the manufacturer or restaurant. This means that to simply multiply fat grams by 9 will often result in a misleading value for percentage of calories from fat.

To more accurately represent the percentage of calories from fat, we developed a simple method called the "compensated 4-4-9 method." Here is how this method was used to calculate the percentage of calories from fat values that appear in this book.

1. We calculated the total calories from each of the calorie sources by

multiplying protein grams by 4, carbohydrate grams by 4, and fat grams by 9. We added these values together to get a "total derived calories" value.

2. We made the assumption that the manufacturer's total calorie value was correct. We then compared our total derived calorie value to the manufacturer's published total calorie value. If our derived value was lower or higher, we adjusted all of the nonzero nutrient values—maintaining the 4-4-9 ratio—to match the manufacturer's total.

3. Using the adjusted nutrient values, we calculated the percentage of calories from fat.

The compensated 4-4-9 method results in percentage-of-calories values for protein, carbohydrates, and fat that both match the manufacturer's total calorie figure and add up to 100 percent of the total calories. Using the nutritional information provided by manufacturers at this time, we feel that this method is the best means of determining accurate values.

We hope you will find *The Nutribase Complete Fast Food Restaurant Nutrition Counter* a valuable companion that provides the information you need to take control of your eating habits. Should you have any comments about this book, feel free to write to the following address: Nutribase Comments, c/o Avery Publishing Group, 120 Old Broadway, Garden City Park, NY 11040.

CODES AND ABBREVIATIONS

To provide the most comprehensive nutritional information possible, a number of codes and abbreviations have been used throughout this book. A complete translation is given below.

>	greater than[1]	(mq)	may contain a measurable quantity [2]
<	less than	na	not available
%	percentage	prot	protein
approx	approximately	raw wt	raw weight
c	crude fiber[1]	sat fat	saturated fat
cal	calcium	sod	sodium
carbs	carbohydrates	tbsp	tablespoon
chol	cholesterol	tr	trace
diam	diameter	(tr)	may contain a trace amount
fl	fluid	tsp	teaspoon
gm	gram	w/	with
lb	pound	w/o	without
mcg	microgram(s)	wt	weight
med	medium-sized		
mgs	milligrams		

[1]The symbols > and c, which are used only in fiber value listings, indicate that the amount

shown is the result of crude analysis, and that the actual amount of fiber present most probably is greater than the amount shown. For further explanation, see page xv.

[2]The food item may contain a quantity ranging from a trace amount to a substantial amount. This quantity depends upon any one of a number of variables—such as soil condition and mineral content of fertilizer used—that may have affected the food item during growing, processing, and/or preparation.

The NutriBase
Complete Fast Food Restaurant
Nutrition Counter

Food Name	Serving Size	Total Calories

ARBY'S

Food Name	Serving Size	Total Calories
AU JUS SAUCE	1 serving	7
BARBECUE SANDWICH, 'Arby Q'	1 serving	389
BEEF SANDWICH		
'Beef'n Cheddar'	1 serving	508
'Philly Beef 'n Swiss'	1 serving	467
BISCUIT, plain	1 serving	280
BREAKFAST		
bacon platter	1 meal	593
'Egg Platter'	1 meal	460
'French Toastix' 3.5 oz	1 serving	420
'Ham Platter'	1 meal	518
'Sausage Platter'	1 meal	640
BREAKFAST SANDWICH		
'Bacon/Egg Croissant'	1 serving	430
biscuit, w/bacon	1 serving	318
'Ham Biscuit'	1 serving	323
'Ham/Cheese Croissant'	1 serving	345
'Sausage Biscuit'	1 serving	460
'Sausage/Egg Croissant'	1 serving	519
BROCCOLI SOUP, cream of	1 serving	166
CATSUP	1 serving	16
CHEESE SOUP, Wisconsin cheese	1 serving	281
CHEESEBURGER, 'Bac'n Cheddar Deluxe'	1 serving	512
CHEESECAKE	1 serving	306
CHICKEN NOODLE SOUP, 'Old Fashioned'	1 serving	99
CHICKEN SANDWICH		
breast, fillet	1 serving	445
cordon bleu	1 serving	518
grilled, barbecue	1 serving	386

Prot. MGS	Carbs. GMS	Sodium MGS	Fiber GMS	Fat GMS	Sat. Fat GMS	Chol. MGS	% Fat Cal.
1.0	1.0	750	na	0.0	0.0	0	0%
17.6	48.2	1268	na	15.2	5.5	29	35%
24.6	43.2	1166	(mq)	26.5	7.7	52	47%
24.1	38.2	1144	na	25.3	9.7	53	49%
6.0	34.0	730	na	14.9	3.3	0	48%
21.8	51.0	880	na	33.0	9.2	458	50%
15.0	44.9	591	na	24.0	7.2	346	47%
8.0	43.0	440	na	25.0	4.6	20	54%
24.4	45.3	1177	na	26.2	7.9	374	46%
21.0	45.9	861	na	41.0	13.3	406	58%
17.4	28.8	720	na	30.0	15.4	245	63%
6.8	35.5	904	na	17.9	4.3	8	51%
13.0	34.3	1169	na	16.6	3.9	21	46%
16.0	29.3	939	na	20.7	12.1	90	54%
12.0	35.0	1000	na	31.9	9.4	60	62%
17.5	29.3	632	na	39.2	18.6	271	68%
7.7	18.0	1050	na	7.2	3.8	24	39%
0.3	4.2	143	na	0.0	0.0	0	0%
9.0	19.7	1084	na	18.0	9.0	32	58%
21.2	38.9	1094	na	31.5	8.7	38	55%
5.2	21.3	220	na	22.8	7.4	95	67%
6.0	14.8	929	na	1.8	0.5	25	16%
22.2	52.1	958	(mq)	22.5	3.0	45	46%
30.0	52.1	1463	na	27.1	5.3	92	47%
23.4	46.7	1002	na	13.1	3.6	43	31%

Food Name	Serving Size	Total Calories
grilled, 'Deluxe'	1 serving	430
roast, 'Club'	1 serving	503
roast, 'Deluxe Light'	1 serving	276
CHOWDER, Boston clam	1 serving	193
COFFEE	8 oz	3
COOKIE, chocolate chip	1 serving	130
CROISSANT, plain	1 serving	260
CROISSANT SANDWICH, 'Mushroom/Cheese'	1 serving	493
CROUTONS	1 serving	59
DANISH, cinnamon nut	1 serving	360
DESSERT		
'Butterfinger Polar Swirl'	1 serving	457
'Heath Polar Swirl'	1 serving	543
'Oreo Polar Swirl'	1 serving	482
'Peanut Butter Cup Polar Swirl'	1 serving	517
'Snickers Polar Swirl'	1 serving	511
FISH SANDWICH, fillet	1 serving	526
FRENCH DIP SANDWICH		
regular	1 serving	368
w/Swiss cheese	1 serving	429
FRENCH FRIES		
cheddar	1 serving	399
curly	1 serving	337
regular, small order, 2.5 oz	1 serving	246
HAM AND CHEESE SANDWICH	1 serving	355
HORSERADISH SAUCE, 'Horsey Sauce'	1 serving	55
HOT CHOCOLATE	8 oz	110
ICED TEA	16 oz	6
MAYONNAISE	1 serving	90
MILK, 2%	8 oz	121
MILKSHAKE		
chocolate	1 serving	451

Prot. MGS	Carbs. GMS	Sodium MGS	Fiber GMS	Fat GMS	Sat. Fat GMS	Chol. MGS	% Fat Cal.
23.6	41.8	901	na	19.9	3.5	44	42%
30.5	36.6	1143	(mq)	27.0	6.9	46	48%
24.0	33.0	777	na	7.0	1.7	33	23%
8.3	17.5	1032	na	10.0	4.5	26	47%
0.0	0.0	3	na	0.0	0.0	0	0%
2.0	17.0	95	na	4.0	2.0	0	28%
6.0	28.0	300	na	15.6	10.4	49	54%
13.0	34.0	935	na	37.7	15.2	116	69%
1.6	8.5	155	na	2.2	0.3	1	34%
6.0	60.0	105	na	11.0	1.0	0	28%
12.1	61.6	318	na	18.1	8.4	28	36%
10.6	76.3	346	na	21.8	5.2	39	36%
10.5	65.8	521	na	19.7	10.4	35	37%
14.0	61.4	385	na	24.0	8.1	34	42%
12.2	73.3	351	na	18.8	6.7	33	33%
23.0	50.0	872	na	27.0	7.0	44	46%
22.0	35.0	1018	na	15.4	5.6	43	38%
28.7	35.5	1438	na	19.0	8.8	67	40%
6.2	46.2	443	na	21.9	9.0	9	49%
4.2	43.2	167	na	17.7	7.4	0	47%
2.1	29.8	114	(mq)	13.2	3.0	0	48%
24.6	34.5	1400	(mq)	14.2	5.1	55	36%
0.1	2.6	105	na	5.0	2.0	0	82%
2.0	23.0	120	na	1.2	0.7	0	10%
0.0	1.0	12	na	0.0	0.0	0	0%
0.0	0.0	75	na	10.0	1.0	0	100%
8.0	12.0	122	na	4.4	3.0	18	33%
10.2	76.5	341	na	11.6	2.8	36	23%

Food Name	Serving Size	Total Calories
jamocha	1 serving	368
vanilla	1 serving	330
MUFFIN, blueberry	1 muffin	240
MUSTARD	1 serving	11
ORANGE JUICE	6 oz	82
POTATO, BAKED		
broccoli and cheddar	1 serving	417
'Deluxe'	1 serving	621
mushroom and cheese	1 serving	515
plain	1 serving	240
w/sour cream and butter	1 serving	463
POTATO CAKES	3 oz	204
POTATO SOUP, w/bacon	1 serving	184
ROAST BEEF SANDWICH		
'Junior'	1 serving	233
'Light Deluxe'	1 serving	294
regular, 5.5 oz	1 serving	383
super	1 serving	552
SALAD		
chef's	1 serving	205
garden	1 serving	117
roast chicken	1 serving	204
side order	1 serving	25
SALAD DRESSING		
blue cheese	1 serving	295
buttermilk ranch	1 serving	349
honey French	1 serving	322
light Italian	1 serving	23
Thousand Island	1 serving	298
SAUCE, Arby's	1 serving	15
SOFT DRINK		
Coca-Cola Classic	12 oz	141
Diet Coke	12 oz	1

Prot. MGS	Carbs. GMS	Sodium MGS	Fiber GMS	Fat GMS	Sat. Fat GMS	Chol. MGS	% Fat Cal.
9.3	59.1	262	na	10.5	2.5	35	26%
10.5	46.2	281	na	11.5	3.9	32	31%
4.0	40.0	200	na	7.0	1.0	22	26%
0.6	0.5	160	na	0.6	0.0	0	49%
1.0	20.0	2	na	0.0	0.0	0	0%
10.5	55.0	361	na	17.9	6.9	22	39%
17.2	58.9	605	na	36.4	18.1	58	53%
15.0	57.5	923	na	26.7	5.8	47	47%
5.8	50.2	58	na	1.9	0.0	0	7%
7.7	52.7	203	na	25.2	12.1	40	49%
1.8	19.8	397	(mq)	12.0	2.2	0	53%
6.5	20.0	1068	na	8.8	4.3	20	43%
11.5	22.8	519	na	10.8	4.1	22	42%
18.0	33.0	826	na	10.0	3.5	42	31%
22.0	35.4	936	(mq)	18.2	7.0	43	43%
23.7	54.1	1174	(mq)	28.3	7.6	43	46%
18.5	13.0	796	na	9.5	3.9	126	42%
7.0	11.4	134	na	5.2	2.7	12	40%
24.0	12.2	508	na	7.2	3.3	43	32%
2.0	4.0	30	na	0.3	0.0	0	11%
2.3	2.5	489	na	31.2	5.8	50	95%
0.3	1.9	471	na	38.5	5.6	6	99%
0.2	21.8	486	na	26.9	3.9	0	75%
0.0	3.5	1110	na	1.1	0.1	0	43%
0.5	9.8	493	na	29.2	4.3	24	88%
0.1	3.3	113	na	0.2	0.0	0	12%
0.0	38.1	15	na	0.0	0.0	0	0%
0.0	0.0	30	na	0.0	0.0	0	0%

Food Name	Serving Size	Total Calories
Diet 7Up	12 oz	4
Nehi Orange	12 oz	190
Pepsi Cola	12 oz	159
R.C. Cola	12 oz	173
R.C. Diet Rite	12 oz	1
R.C. Root Beer	12 oz	173
7Up	12 oz	144
Upper Ten	12 oz	169
SUBMARINE SANDWICH		
Italian	1 serving	671
roast beef	1 serving	623
tuna	1 serving	663
turkey	1 serving	486
SUGAR SUBSTITUTE	1 serving	4
SYRUP, maple, 1.5 oz	1 serving	120
TURKEY SANDWICH, 'Light Roast Turkey Deluxe' 6.8 oz	1 serving	260
TURNOVER		
apple	1 serving	303
blueberry	1 serving	320
cherry	1 serving	280
VEGETABLE SOUP, mixed vegetable, 'Lumberjack'	1 serving	89

ARTHUR TREACHER'S

CHICKEN PATTIES, 4.8 oz	2 patties	369
CHICKEN SANDWICH, 5.5 oz	1 serving	413
COD FILLET, tail shape, 'Bake'n Broil' 5 oz	1 serving	245
COLESLAW, 3 oz	1 serving	123
DESSERT, 'Lemon Luv' 3 oz	1 serving	276
FISH, 5.2 oz	2 pieces	355

Prot. MGS	Carbs. GMS	Sodium MGS	Fiber GMS	Fat GMS	Sat. Fat GMS	Chol. MGS	% Fat Cal.
0.3	0.0	22	na	0.0	0.0	0	0%
0.0	47.4	21	na	0.0	0.0	0	0%
0.0	40.0	10	na	0.0	0.0	0	0%
0.0	43.2	1	na	0.0	0.0	0	0%
0.0	0.2	10	na	0.0	0.0	0	0%
0.0	42.9	16	na	0.0	0.0	0	0%
0.0	38.0	34	na	0.0	0.0	0	0%
0.0	42.3	40	na	0.0	0.0	0	0%
34.1	47.4	2062	na	38.8	12.8	69	52%
37.7	46.8	1847	na	32.0	11.5	73	46%
74.0	50.2	1342	na	37.0	8.2	43	50%
32.8	46.5	2033	na	19.0	5.3	51	35%
0.0	0.0	5	na	0.0	0.0	0	0%
0.0	29.0	52	na	0.1	0.0	0	1%
20.0	33.0	1262	na	6.0	1.6	33	21%
4.4	27.5	178	na	18.3	6.9	0	54%
3.0	32.0	240	na	19.0	6.3	0	53%
4.6	25.4	200	na	17.8	5.3	0	57%
2.3	12.6	1075	na	3.6	1.7	4	36%
27.1	16.5	495	(mq)	21.6	3.5	65	53%
16.2	44.0	708	(mq)	19.2	2.8	32	42%
19.6	9.7	144	(mq)	14.2	(mq)	(mq)	52%
1.0	11.1	266	(mq)	8.2	1.1	7	60%
2.6	35.1	314	(mq)	13.9	2.2	<1	45%
19.2	25.4	450	(mq)	19.8	2.8	56	50%

Food Name	Serving Size	Total Calories
FISH SANDWICH, 5.5 oz	1 serving	440
FRENCH FRIES, 'Chips' 4 oz	1 serving	276
HUSHPUPPY, 'Krunch Pup' 2 oz	1 piece	203
SHRIMP, 4.1 oz	7 pieces	381

AU BON PAIN

BAGEL		
cinnamon	1 bagel	395
onion	1 bagel	390
plain	1 bagel	380
sesame	1 bagel	425
BEEF BARLEY SOUP		
bowl	1 serving	112
cup	1 serving	75
BREAD		
baguette	1 loaf	810
cheese	1 loaf	1670
four grain	1 loaf	1420
onion herb	1 loaf	1430
pita pocket	2 slices	80
Ponsienne	1 loaf	1490
sandwich, multigrain	2 slices	391
sandwich, rye	2 slices	374
BROCCOLI SOUP, CREAM OF		
bowl	1 serving	302
cup	1 serving	201
CHEESE		
boursin, sandwich filling	1 serving	290
brie, sandwich filling	1 serving	300
cheddar, sandwich filling	1 serving	110
provolone, sandwich filling	1 serving	155
Swiss, sandwich filling	1 serving	330

Prot. MGS	Carbs. GMS	Sodium MGS	Fiber GMS	Fat GMS	Sat. Fat GMS	Chol. MGS	% Fat Cal.
16.4	39.4	836	(mq)	24.0	4.2	42	49%
4.0	34.9	39	(mq)	13.2	2.3	5	43%
5.4	12.0	446	(mq)	14.8	3.7	25	66%
13.1	27.2	538	(mq)	24.4	3.3	93	58%
14.0	86.0	605	4.0	2.0	<1.0	0	5%
16.0	81.0	665	4.0	2.0	<1.0	0	5%
15.0	79.0	665	3.0	2.0	<1.0	0	5%
17.0	81.0	665	4.0	5.0	1.0	0	11%
9.0	15.0	901	na	3.0	na	18	24%
6.0	10.0	600	na	2.0	na	12	24%
27.0	166.0	1830	na	2.0	<1.0	0	2%
70.0	269.0	4140	na	29.0	9.0	75	16%
57.0	262.0	3050	na	11.0	<1.0	1	7%
52.0	263.0	2390	na	13.0	<1.0	0	8%
2.7	18.0	na	na	<1.0	na	na	0%
49.0	166.0	3380	na	4.0	<1.0	0	2%
16.0	77.0	2040	na	3.0	1.0	1	7%
14.0	73.0	2170	na	4.0	1.0	na	10%
8.0	18.0	219	na	26.0	12.0	54	77%
5.0	12.0	146	na	17.0	8.0	36	76%
6.0	2.0	390	na	29.0	18.0	90	90%
18.0	3.0	510	na	24.0	15.0	85	72%
7.0	1.0	150	na	9.0	5.0	30	74%
9.9	<1.0	180	na	12.6	7.4	36	73%
25.0	3.0	230	na	24.0	15.0	80	65%

Food Name	Serving Size	Total Calories
CHICKEN NOODLE SOUP		
bowl	1 serving	119
cup	1 serving	79
CHICKEN POT PIE	1 serving	440
CHICKEN SANDWICH		
cracked pepper, on French roll	1 sandwich	440
cracked pepper, on hearth roll	1 sandwich	490
cracked pepper, on soft roll	1 sandwich	430
grilled, on French roll	1 sandwich	450
grilled, on hearth roll	1 sandwich	500
grilled, on soft roll	1 sandwich	440
tarragon, on French roll	1 sandwich	590
tarragon, on hearth roll	1 sandwich	640
tarragon, on soft roll	1 sandwich	580
CHILI, VEGETARIAN		
bowl	1 serving	208
cup	1 serving	139
CHOWDER, clam		
bowl	1 serving	433
cup	1 serving	289
COOKIE		
chocolate chip, 'Gourmet'	1 cookie	280
chocolate chunk pecan, 'Gourmet'	1 cookie	290
oatmeal raisin, 'Gourmet'	1 cookie	250
peanut butter, 'Gourmet'	1 cookie	290
shortbread, 'Gourmet'	1 cookie	425
white chocolate chunk pecan, 'Gourmet'	1 cookie	300
CROISSANT		
almond	1 croissant	420
apple	1 croissant	250
blueberry cheese	1 croissant	380
chocolate	1 croissant	400
cinnamon raisin	1 croissant	390

Prot. MGS	Carbs. GMS	Sodium MGS	Fiber GMS	Fat GMS	Sat. Fat GMS	Chol. MGS	% Fat Cal.
12.0	14.0	743	na	1.7	<1.0	26	13%
8.0	9.0	495	na	1.0	<1.0	17	11%
17.5	46.0	1109	na	21.0	7.0	45	43%
33.0	66.0	1390	na	3.0	na	50	6%
39.0	70.0	1280	na	5.0	na	50	9%
31.0	51.0	1090	na	10.0	na	50	21%
33.0	66.0	1320	na	5.0	na	60	10%
39.0	70.0	1210	na	7.0	na	60	13%
31.0	51.0	1020	na	12.0	na	60	25%
34.0	68.0	1014	na	16.0	na	70	24%
40.0	72.0	904	na	18.0	na	70	25%
32.0	53.0	714	na	23.0	na	70	36%
9.0	37.0	763	na	4.0	<1.0	0	17%
6.0	24.0	508	na	3.0	<1.0	0	19%
17.0	36.0	1029	na	27.0	15.0	90	56%
11.0	24.0	687	na	18.0	9.0	60	56%
2.0	37.0	70	na	15.0	9.0	25	48%
3.0	37.0	200	na	17.0	6.0	10	53%
4.0	41.0	230	na	9.0	na	10	32%
7.0	33.0	250	na	15.0	6.0	10	47%
5.0	46.0	385	na	26.0	16.0	68	55%
3.0	37.0	200	na	17.0	6.0	10	51%
8.0	41.0	250	na	25.0	12.0	95	54%
4.0	38.0	150	na	10.0	6.0	25	36%
7.0	44.0	280	na	20.0	12.0	60	47%
5.0	46.0	220	na	24.0	14.0	35	54%
7.0	60.0	240	na	13.0	8.0	35	30%

Food Name	Serving Size	Total Calories
coconut pecan	1 croissant	440
hazelnut chocolate	1 croissant	480
hot, filled w/ham and cheese	1 serving	370
hot, filled w/spinach and cheese	1 serving	290
hot, filled w/turkey and cheddar	1 serving	410
hot, filled w/turkey and havarti	1 serving	410
plain	1 croissant	220
raspberry cheese	1 croissant	400
strawberry cheese	1 croissant	400
sweet cheese	1 croissant	420
DANISH PASTRY		
cheese	1 Danish	390
cherry	1 Danish	335
cherry dumpling	1 Danish	360
raspberry	1 Danish	335
HAM SANDWICH		
country ham, on French roll	1 sandwich	470
country ham, on hearth roll	1 sandwich	520
country ham, on soft roll	1 sandwich	460
MINESTRONE SOUP, cup	1 serving	105
MUFFIN		
blueberry, gourmet	1 muffin	390
bran, gourmet	1 muffin	390
carrot, gourmet	1 muffin	450
corn, gourmet	1 muffin	460
cranberry walnut, gourmet	1 muffin	350
oat bran apple, gourmet	1 muffin	400
pumpkin, gourmet	1 muffin	410
whole grain, gourmet	1 muffin	440
ROAST BEEF SANDWICH		
on French roll	1 sandwich	500
on hearth roll	1 sandwich	550
on soft roll	1 sandwich	490

Prot. MGS	Carbs. GMS	Sodium MGS	Fiber GMS	Fat GMS	Sat. Fat GMS	Chol. MGS	% Fat Cal.
7.0	51.0	290	na	23.0	12.0	45	47%
6.0	56.0	220	na	28.0	14.0	35	53%
10.0	38.0	280	na	20.0	12.0	55	49%
9.0	29.0	310	na	16.0	10.0	45	50%
16.0	38.0	680	na	22.0	13.0	70	48%
17.0	38.0	630	na	21.0	13.0	70	46%
5.0	29.0	240	na	10.0	6.0	25	41%
7.0	49.0	280	na	20.0	12.0	60	45%
7.0	49.0	280	na	20.0	12.0	60	45%
8.0	45.0	310	na	23.0	14.0	70	49%
8.0	43.0	530	2.0	22.0	12.0	78	51%
7.0	42.0	480	2.0	16.0	8.0	50	43%
5.0	59.0	255	1.0	13.0	2.0	0	33%
6.0	43.0	480	2.0	16.0	8.0	50	43%
27.0	68.0	1680	na	8.0	na	115	15%
33.0	72.0	1570	na	10.0	na	115	17%
25.0	53.0	1380	na	15.0	na	115	29%
5.0	20.0	265	na	2.0	na	1	17%
8.0	66.0	410	na	4.0	na	40	9%
7.0	73.0	940	na	11.0	na	20	25%
7.0	58.0	610	na	22.0	5.0	15	44%
8.0	71.0	510	na	17.0	3.0	25	33%
7.0	53.0	730	na	13.0	na	15	33%
7.0	71.0	590	na	2.0	na	0	5%
6.0	63.0	500	na	16.0	2.0	20	35%
10.0	68.0	310	na	16.0	2.0	30	33%
34.0	66.0	1020	na	9.0	na	60	16%
40.0	70.0	910	na	11.0	na	60	18%
32.0	51.0	720	na	16.0	na	60	29%

Food Name	Serving Size	Total Calories
ROLL		
Alpine, fresh	1 roll	220
country seed, fresh	1 roll	220
hearth, fresh	1 roll	250
'Petit Pain' fresh	1 roll	220
pumpernickel, fresh	1 roll	210
rye, fresh	1 roll	230
sandwich, braided	1 roll	387
sandwich, croissant	1 roll	300
sandwich, French	1 roll	320
sandwich, hearth	1 roll	370
sandwich, soft	1 roll	310
3 seed raisin, fresh	1 roll	250
vegetable, fresh	1 roll	230
SALAD		
garden, chicken tarragon	1 serving	310
garden, cracked pepper chicken	1 serving	100
garden, grilled chicken	1 serving	110
garden, large	1 serving	40
garden, shrimp	1 serving	102
garden, small	1 serving	20
garden, tuna	1 serving	350
Italian, low-calorie	1 serving	68
SPLIT PEA SOUP		
bowl	1 serving	264
cup	1 serving	176
TOMATO SOUP, Florentine		
bowl	1 serving	92
cup	1 serving	61
TURKEY SANDWICH		
smoked turkey, on French roll	1 sandwich	420
smoked turkey, on hearth roll	1 sandwich	470
smoked turkey, on soft roll	1 sandwich	410

Prot. MGS	Carbs. GMS	Sodium MGS	Fiber GMS	Fat GMS	Sat. Fat GMS	Chol. MGS	% Fat Cal.
8.0	43.0	810	na	3.0	na	0	12%
9.0	37.0	460	na	4.0	na	0	16%
10.0	42.0	510	na	2.0	na	0	7%
7.0	44.0	490	na	<1.0	na	0	0%
8.0	42.0	1005	na	2.0	na	0	9%
8.0	44.0	na	na	2.0	na	0	8%
10.0	64.0	1540	na	11.0	3.0	34	26%
7.0	38.0	240	na	14.0	8.0	35	42%
10.0	65.0	710	na	<1.0	na	0	0%
16.0	69.0	600	na	3.0	na	0	7%
8.0	50.0	410	na	8.0	na	0	23%
8.0	46.0	480	na	4.0	na	0	14%
6.0	40.0	410	na	5.0	na	0	20%
24.0	11.0	332	na	15.0	na	70	44%
14.0	9.0	360	na	2.0	na	25	18%
14.0	9.0	330	na	2.0	na	30	16%
3.0	8.0	20	na	<1.0	<1.0	0	0%
11.0	8.0	193	na	2.0	na	105	18%
5.0	5.0	10	na	<1.0	na	0	0%
21.0	11.0	480	na	25.0	4.0	40	64%
0.0	3.0	360	na	6.0	na	5	79%
18.0	45.0	453	na	2.0	na	1	7%
12.0	30.0	303	na	1.0	na	1	5%
4.0	15.0	221	na	1.7	<1.0	0	17%
3.0	10.0	147	na	1.0	<1.0	0	15%
32.0	65.0	1660	na	2.0	na	35	4%
38.0	69.0	1550	na	4.0	na	35	8%
30.0	50.0	1360	na	9.0	na	35	20%

Food Name	Serving Size	Total Calories
VEGETARIAN SOUP, garden		
bowl .... 1 serving		44
cup .... 1 serving		29

BASKIN ROBBINS

ICE CREAM

'Almond Buttercrunch' light .... 1 serving		130
'Caramel Banana' fat-free .... 1 serving		100
'Chocolate' .... 1 scoop		270
'Chocolate Caramel Nut' light .... 1/2 cup		130
'Chocolate Chip' .... 1 scoop		260
'Chocolate Chip' sugar-free .... 1 serving		100
'Chocolate Raspberry Truffle' .... 1 scoop		310
'Chocolate Wonder' fat-free .... 1 serving		120
'Chunky Banana' sugar-free .... 1/2 cup		100
'Double Raspberry' light .... 1 serving		120
'Expresso and Cream' light .... 1/2 cup		120
'French Vanilla' .... 1 scoop		280
'Jamocha Almond Fudge' .... 1 scoop		270
'Just Chocolate Vanilla' fat-free .... 1/2 cup		100
'Just Peachy' fat-free .... 1/2 cup		100
'Praline Dream' light .... 1/2 cup		130
'Pralines 'N Cream' .... 1 scoop		280
'Rocky Road' .... 1 scoop		300
'Strawberry Royal,' light .... 1/2 cup		110
'Strawberry' sugar-free .... 1 serving		80
'Vanilla' .... 1 scoop		240
'Very Berry Strawberry' .... 1 scoop		220
'World Class Chocolate' .... 1 scoop		280

ICE CREAM BAR

chocolate, caramel ribbon,		
'Sundae Bars' light .... 1 bar		150

Prot. MGS	Carbs. GMS	Sodium MGS	Fiber GMS	Fat GMS	Sat. Fat GMS	Chol. MGS	% Fat Cal.
1.7	9.0	92	na	<1.0	<1.0	0	0%
1.0	6.0	61	na	<1.0	<1.0	0	0%
3.0	16.0	na	na	6.0	na	12	42%
2.0	23.0	na	na	0.0	na	1	0%
5.0	32.0	160	na	14.0	na	37	47%
3.0	19.0	0	na	5.0	3.0	8	35%
4.0	27.0	110	na	15.0	na	40	52%
3.0	20.0	na	na	2.0	na	4	18%
4.0	35.0	115	na	17.0	na	45	49%
3.0	26.0	na	na	0.0	na	1	0%
3.0	20.0	50	na	1.0	na	3	9%
2.0	19.0	na	na	4.0	na	9	30%
3.0	15.0	0	na	5.0	3.0	12	38%
4.0	25.0	90	na	18.0	na	90	58%
5.0	30.0	115	na	14.0	na	32	47%
4.0	21.0	60	na	0.0	na	0	0%
3.0	22.0	60	na	0.0	na	0	0%
3.0	17.0	85	na	6.0	na	11	42%
4.0	35.0	180	na	14.0	na	36	45%
5.0	39.0	135	na	14.0	na	32	42%
2.0	19.0	120	na	3.0	na	9	25%
2.0	17.0	70	na	1.0	na	3	11%
4.0	24.0	115	na	14.0	na	52	53%
3.0	30.0	95	na	10.0	na	30	41%
5.0	35.0	145	na	14.0	na	36	45%
3.0	24.0	75	na	5.0	na	11	30%

Food Name	Serving Size	Total Calories
ICE CREAM CONE		
sugar	1 cone	60
waffle	1 cone	140
SHERBET/SORBET		
daiquiri ice	1 scoop	140
fruit whip sorbet	1 serving	80
rainbow sherbet	1 scoop	160
red raspberry sorbet	1 scoop	140
strawberry soft-serve sorbet	1 serving	100
YOGURT, FROZEN		
cafe mocha, 'Trulyfree'	1 serving	70
chocolate, low-fat, large	9 oz	315
chocolate, low-fat, medium	7 oz	246
chocolate, low-fat, small	5 oz	175
coconut, nonfat, large	9 oz	180
coconut, nonfat, medium	7 oz	140
coconut, nonfat, small	5 oz	100
raspberry, nonfat, large	9 oz	225
raspberry, nonfat, medium	7 oz	164
raspberry, nonfat, small	5 oz	125
strawberry, low-fat, large	9 oz	270
strawberry, low-fat, medium	7 oz	211
strawberry, low-fat, small	5 oz	150
strawberry, nonfat, large	9 oz	225
strawberry, nonfat, medium	7 oz	176
strawberry, nonfat, small	5 oz	125
vanilla, low-fat, large	9 oz	270
vanilla, low-fat, medium	7 oz	211
vanilla, low-fat, small	5 oz	150

BEN & JERRY'S

Aztec harvest coffee	1/2 cup	230

Prot. MGS	Carbs. GMS	Sodium MGS	Fiber GMS	Fat GMS	Sat. Fat GMS	Chol. MGS	% Fat Cal.
1.0	11.0	45	na	1.0	na	0	15%
3.0	28.0	5	na	2.0	na	0	13%
0.0	35.0	15	na	0.0	0.0	0	0%
0.0	24.0	20	na	0.0	0.0	0	0%
1.0	34.0	85	na	2.0	na	6	11%
0.0	34.0	25	na	0.0	0.0	0	0%
0.0	20.0	20	na	0.0	na	0	0%
4.0	16.0	14	na	0.0	0.0	0	0%
9.0	54.0	90	na	9.0	na	9	26%
7.0	42.0	70	na	7.0	na	7	26%
5.0	30.0	50	na	5.0	na	5	26%
9.0	45.0	90	na	0.0	na	0	0%
7.0	35.0	70	na	0.0	na	0	0%
5.0	25.0	50	na	0.0	na	0	0%
9.0	45.0	90	na	0.0	na	0	0%
7.0	35.0	70	na	0.0	na	0	0%
5.0	25.0	50	na	0.0	na	0	0%
9.0	54.0	90	na	9.0	na	9	30%
7.0	42.0	70	na	7.0	na	7	30%
5.0	30.0	50	na	5.0	na	5	30%
9.0	45.0	90	na	0.0	na	0	0%
7.0	35.0	70	na	0.0	na	0	0%
5.0	25.0	50	na	0.0	na	0	0%
9.0	54.0	90	na	9.0	na	9	30%
7.0	42.0	70	na	7.0	na	7	30%
5.0	30.0	50	na	5.0	na	5	30%
4.0	22.0	55	0	16.0	10.0	90	63%

Food Name	Serving Size	Total Calories
Butter pecan	1/2 cup	310
'Cherry Garcia'	1/2 cup	240
Chocolate chip cookie dough	1/2 cup	270
'Chocolate Fudge Brownie'	1/2 cup	250
Chocolate peanut butter cookie dough	1/2 cup	300
'Chunky Monkey' banana	1/2 cup	280
Coconut almond fudge chip	1/2 cup	320
'Coffee Toffee Crunch'	1/2 cup	280
Deep dark chocolate	1/2 cup	260
Double chocolate fudge	1/2 cup	280
Mint with chocolate cookie	1/2 cup	260
Mocha fudge	1/2 cup	270
'New York Super Fudge Chunk'	1/2 cup	290
'Rainforest crunch' vanilla	1/2 cup	300
Vanilla	1/2 cup	230
Vanilla bean	1/2 cup	230
Vanilla caramel fudge	1/2 cup	280
'Wavy Gravy' vanilla crunch	1/2 cup	330
White Russian	1/2 cup	240

BIG BOY RESTAURANT

BEANS, green	1 serving	28
CABBAGE SOUP		
bowl	1 serving	43
cup	1 serving	37
CARROTS	1 serving	35
CHICKEN DINNER		
breast, salad w/o dressing, oat bran bread	1 serving	349
breast, w/mozzarella, salad w/o dressing, bread	1 serving	370

Prot. MGS	Carbs. GMS	Sodium MGS	Fiber GMS	Fat GMS	Sat. Fat GMS	Chol. MGS	% Fat Cal.
4.0	20.0	160	1.0	26.0	11.0	100	75%
4.0	25.0	60	0	16.0	10.0	80	60%
4.0	30.0	92	0	17.0	9.0	80	57%
4.0	31.0	100	2.0	14.0	9.0	50	50%
6.0	32.0	85	2.0	20.0	9.0	55	60%
4.0	29.0	50	1.0	19.0	10.0	70	61%
6.0	24.0	82	2.0	28.0	15.0	75	79%
4.0	28.0	120	0	19.0	10.0	80	61%
4.0	32.0	55	2.0	15.0	9.0	55	52%
5.0	35.0	60	3.0	16.0	9.0	55	51%
4.0	27.0	120	1.0	17.0	10.0	80	59%
5.0	30.0	65	1.0	18.0	10.0	85	60%
5.0	28.0	55	2.0	20.0	11.0	50	62%
5.0	24.0	140	0	23.0	11.0	85	69%
4.0	21.0	55	0	17.0	10.0	95	67%
4.0	21.0	55	0	17.0	10.0	95	67%
4.0	33.0	75	1.0	17.0	10.0	95	55%
6.0	29.0	95	2.0	24.0	10.0	80	65%
4.0	23.0	55	0	16.0	10.0	90	60%
2.0	6.0	1	na	0.0	0.0	0	0%
2.0	9.0	727	na	1.0	na	1	21%
2.0	8.0	623	na	0.0	0.0	1	0%
1.0	8.0	38	na	0.0	0.0	0	0%
38.0	20.0	342	na	13.0	na	65	34%
42.0	24.0	353	na	12.0	na	76	29%

Food Name	Serving Size	Total Calories
Cajun, salad w/o dressing, oat bran bread	1 serving	349
chicken and vegetable stir-fry	1 serving	562
CHICKEN SANDWICH, pita, w/mozzarella, 'Heart Smart'	1 serving	404
CORN	1 serving	90
DESSERT, 'No-no' frozen dessert	1 serving	75
FISH DINNER		
cod, baked, Dijon, salad w/o dressing, oat bran bread	1 serving	427
cod, baked, salad w/o dressing, oat bran bread	1 serving	364
cod, broiled, Dijon, salad w/o dressing, oat bran bread	1 serving	427
cod, broiled, salad w/o dressing, oat bran bread	1 serving	364
cod, Cajun, salad w/o dressing, oat bran bread	1 serving	364
MIXED VEGETABLES	1 serving	27
PEAS	1 serving	77
POTATO, BAKED	1 serving	163
RICE	1 serving	114
ROLL	1 roll	139
SALAD		
chicken breast, Dijon	1 serving	391
dinner, w/o dressing	1 serving	19
SALAD DRESSING, buttermilk	1 serving	36
SPAGHETTI DINNER		
marinara, salad w/o dressing, oat bran bread	1 serving	450
TURKEY SANDWICH, pita, 'Heart Smart'	1 serving	224
VEGETABLE STIR-FRY	1 serving	408

Prot. MGS	Carbs. GMS	Sodium MGS	Fiber GMS	Fat GMS	Sat. Fat GMS	Chol. MGS	% Fat Cal.
38.0	20.0	612	na	13.0	na	65	34%
43.0	68.0	750	na	14.0	na	68	22%
42.0	26.0	421	na	13.0	na	76	29%
3.0	21.0	1	na	1.0	na	0	10%
2.0	17.0	36	na	0.0	0.0	0	0%
44.0	21.0	567	na	18.0	na	68	38%
43.0	20.0	371	na	12.0	na	68	30%
44.0	21.0	567	na	18.0	na	68	38%
43.0	20.0	371	na	12.0	na	68	30%
43.0	20.0	461	na	12.0	na	68	30%
2.0	5.0	42	na	0.0	0.0	0	0%
6.0	13.0	131	na	0.0	0.0	0	0%
5.0	37.0	7	na	0.0	0.0	0	0%
3.0	25.0	633	na	0.0	0.0	0	0%
3.0	30.0	187	na	0.0	0.0	2	0%
42.0	31.0	415	na	11.0	na	65	25%
1.0	4.0	11	na	0.0	na	0	0%
0.0	4.0	151	na	2.0	na	10	50%
15.0	87.0	761	na	6.0	na	8	12%
22.0	24.0	833	na	5.0	na	75	20%
9.0	74.0	703	na	10.0	na	0	22%

Food Name	Serving Size	Total Calories
YOGURT, FROZEN		
regular	1 serving	72
shake	1 serving	184

BOJANGLES

BISCUIT	1 serving	239
CHICKEN		
breast, skin-free, 'Southern'	4 oz	271
leg, skin-free, 'Southern'	1.8 oz	128
thigh, skin-free, 'Southern'	3.2 oz	264
CHICKEN SANDWICH, fillet, grilled,		
w/o mayonnaise	1 serving	329
COLESLAW	1 serving	105
PINTO BEANS, Cajun	1 serving	124
RICE, 'Dirty'	1 serving	167

BONANZA RESTAURANTS

HALIBUT, fillet	6 oz	139
RIB EYE STEAK	5.5 oz	196

BOSTON MARKET (formerly BOSTON CHICKEN)

APPLES, cinnamon, hot	3/4 cup	250
BAKED BEANS, barbecue	3/4 cup	330
BROWNIE	1 brownie	450
CAESAR SALAD		
chicken	13 oz	670
entree	10 oz	520
side	4 oz	210
w/o dressing	8 oz	240

Prot. MGS	Carbs. GMS	Sodium MGS	Fiber GMS	Fat GMS	Sat. Fat GMS	Chol. MGS	% Fat Cal.
2.0	16.0	31	na	0.0	0.0	0	0%
8.0	36.0	127	na	0.0	na	2	0%
4.0	30.0	588	na	11.0	na	1	41%
28.0	11.0	869	na	13.0	na	104	43%
7.0	5.0	312	na	12.0	na	54	84%
19.0	10.0	592	na	17.0	na	88	58%
27.0	37.0	418	na	7.0	na	59	19%
1.0	19.0	406	na	4.0	na	0	34%
6.0	25.0	463	na	0.0	na	0	0%
5.0	21.0	397	na	7.0	na	12	38%
26.0	3.0	128	na	2.0	na	60	13%
28.0	1.0	563	na	8.0	na	50	37%
0	53	45	3.0	4.5	0.5	0	16%
11.0	53.0	630	9.0	9.0	3.0	10	24%
6.0	47.0	190	3.0	27.0	7.0	80	53%
45.0	16.0	1860	3.0	47.0	13.0	120	18%
20.0	16.0	1420	3.0	43.0	12.0	40	75%
8.0	6.0	560	1.0	17.0	4.5	20	71%
19.0	14.0	780	3.0	13.0	7.0	25	50%

Food Name	Serving Size	Total Calories
CHICKEN		
1/2 chicken, w/skin	10.18 oz	630
1/4 chicken, dark meat, w/skin	4.71 oz	330
1/4 chicken, dark meat, w/o skin	3.71 oz	210
1/4 chicken, white meat, w/skin	5.46 oz	330
1/4 chicken, white meat, w/o skin	3.71 oz	160
CHICKEN ENTRÉE		
1/4 chicken, white meat, corn bread, corn, new potatoes	15.8 oz	690
1/4 chicken, white meat, corn bread, cranberry, new potatoes	18.6 oz	870
1/4 chicken, white meat, corn bread, vegetables, corn	15.0 oz	590
1/4 chicken, white meat, corn bread, vegetables, fruit	15.3 oz	470
CHICKEN GRAVY	1 oz	15
CHICKEN POT PIE, 15 oz	1 pie	750
CHICKEN SALAD, chunky	3/4 cup	390
CHICKEN SANDWICH		
breast, 9.1 oz	1 sandwich	420
breast, w/fruit salad, 14.6 oz	1 sandwich	490
chunky chicken salad, 10.8 oz	1 sandwich	640
CHICKEN SOUP	3/4 cup	80
CHICKEN SOUP ENTRÉE		
w/corn bread, steamed vegetables, new potatoes	17.5 oz	470
CHOCOLATE CHIP COOKIE, 2.8 oz	1 cookie	340
COLESLAW	3/4 cup	280
CORN, buttered	3/4 cup	190
CORNBREAD, 2.4 oz	1 loaf	200
CRANBERRY RELISH	3/4 cup	370
CUCUMBER SALAD	4.79 oz	79
FRUIT SALAD	3/4 cup	70

Prot. MGS	Carbs. GMS	Sodium MGS	Fiber GMS	Fat GMS	Sat. Fat GMS	Chol. MGS	% Fat Cal.
74.0	370	960	0	37.0	19.0	370	52%
31.0	2.0	460	0	22.0	6.0	180	61%
28.0	1.0	320	0	10.0	2.5	150	43%
43.0	2.0	530	0	17.0	4.5	175	45%
31.0	0.0	350	0	4.0	1.0	95	22%
na	na	970	na	17.0	4.0	120	22%
na	na	850	na	18.0	3.5	120	18%
na	na	910	na	15.0	3.5	120	22%
na	na	790	na	11.0	2.5	120	20%
0	2.0	170	0	1.0	0	0	67%
34.0	78.0	2380	6.0	34.0	9.0	115	40%
27.0	3.0	790	1.0	30.0	5.0	145	69%
41.0	50.0	900	4.0	5.0	1.0	100	11%
na	na	910	na	6.0	1.0	100	10%
37.0	53.0	1330	5.0	31.0	5.0	145	44%
9.0	4.0	470	1.0	3.0	1.0	25	31%
na	na	790	na	11.0	2.5	120	20%
4.0	48.0	240	1.0	17.0	6.0	25	44%
2.0	32.0	520	3.0	16.0	2.5	25	50%
6.0	39.0	130	4.0	4.0	1.0	0	18%
3.0	33.0	390	1.0	6.0	1.5	25	25%
2.0	84.0	5.0	5.0	5.0	0.5	0	12%
1.0	4.0	182	1.0	6.5	1.0	1	74%
1.0	17.0	10.0	2.0	0.5	0	0	7%

Food Name	Serving Size	Total Calories
MACARONI AND CHEESE	3/4 cup	280
OATMEAL RAISIN COOKIE, 2.8 oz	1 loaf	320
PASTA SALAD		
Mediterranean	3/4 cup	170
tortellini	3/4 cup	380
POTATOES		
mashed	2/3 cup	180
mashed, homemade, w/gravy	3/4 cup	200
new	3/4 cup	140
RICE PILAF	2/3 cup	180
SPINACH, creamed	3/4 cup	300
SQUASH, butternut	3/4 cup	160
STUFFING	3/4 cup	310
TURKEY		
breast, skinless	5.07 oz	170
breast, skinless w/gravy	8.11 oz	200
sandwich w/o mayo or mustard	9.39 oz	440
VEGETABLE POT PIE, 17 oz	1 pie	350
VEGETABLES, steamed	2/3 cup	35
ZUCCHINI, marinara	3/4 cup	80

BRAUM'S

YOGURT, FROZEN		
diet, sugar-free w/NutraSweet	1 serving	90
fat-free	1 serving	90
regular	1 serving	180

BRESLER'S

ICE CREAM, 'Royal Lites' all flavors . . .	1 serving	132
SHERBET, all flavors	1 serving	160

Prot. MGS	Carbs. GMS	Sodium MGS	Fiber GMS	Fat GMS	Sat. Fat GMS	Chol. MGS	% Fat Cal.
12.0	36.0	760	1.0	10.0	9.0	20	32%
4.0	48.0	260	1.0	6.0	2.5	25	34%
4.0	16.0	490	2.0	10.0	2.5	10	53%
14.0	29.0	530	2.0	24.0	4.5	90	59%
3.0	25.0	390	2.0	8.0	5.0	25	44%
3.0	27.0	560	2.0	9.0	5.0	25	40%
3.0	25.0	100	2.0	3.0	0.5	0	18%
5.0	32.0	600	2.0	5.0	1.0	0	25%
10.0	13.0	790	2.0	24.0	15.0	75	73%
2.0	25.0	580	3.0	6.0	4.0	15	38%
6.0	44.0	1140	3.0	12.0	2.0	0	35%
36.0	1.0	850	0	1.0	0.5	100	6%
37.0	7.0	1370	0	3.5	1.0	100	15%
38.0	53	1130	4	8.0	4.5	80	16%
12.0	52.0	1450	7.0	12.0	7.0	35	31%
2.0	7.0	35	3.0	0.5	0	0	14%
2.0	10.0	470	2.0	4.0	0.5	0	50%
3.0	13.0	na	na	3.0	na	na	30%
4.0	20.0	55	na	0.0	na	na	0%
3.0	16.0	35	na	3.0	na	na	15%
5.0	9.0	70	na	5.0	na	16	34%
1.0	34.0	na	na	2.0	na	6	11%

Food Name	Serving Size	Total Calories

YOGURT, FROZEN
| gourmet, all flavors | 1 serving | 116 |
| lite, all flavors | 1 serving | 108 |

BURGER CHEF

APPLE TURNOVER	1 serving	237

BREAKFAST
scrambled eggs and bacon platter	1 serving	567
scrambled eggs and sausage platter	1 serving	668
w/bacon, 'Sunrise'	1 serving	392
w/sausage, 'Sunrise'	1 serving	526

BREAKFAST SANDWICH,
| sausage biscuit | 1 serving | 418 |

CHEESEBURGER
double	1 serving	402
regular	1 serving	278
CLUB SANDWICH, chicken	1 serving	521
FISH SANDWICH, 'Fisherman's Fillet'	1 serving	534

FRENCH FRIES
| large order | 1 serving | 285 |
| regular order | 1 serving | 204 |

HAMBURGER
'Big Chef'	1 serving	556
mushroom	1 serving	520
regular	1 serving	235
'Super Chef'	1 serving	604
'Top Chef'	1 serving	541
HAMBURGER MEAL, 'Funmeal'	1 serving	514

MILKSHAKE
| chocolate | 1 serving | 403 |
| vanilla | 1 serving | 380 |

Prot. MGS	Carbs. GMS	Sodium MGS	Fiber GMS	Fat GMS	Sat. Fat GMS	Chol. MGS	% Fat Cal.
4.0	22.0	na	na	2.0	na	7	16%
4.0	24.0	na	na	0.0	0.0	0	0%
2.0	38.0	na	na	9.0	na	na	34%
21.0	50.0	1108	na	31.0	na	na	49%
26.0	50.0	1411	na	40.0	na	479	54%
19.0	30.0	978	na	21.0	na	384	48%
26.0	30.0	1412	na	33.0	na	419	56%
16.0	33.0	1313	na	25.0	na	45	54%
23.0	28.0	835	na	22.0	na	74	49%
14.0	28.0	641	na	12.0	na	37	39%
36.0	33.0	na	na	25.0	na	na	43%
26.0	41.0	na	na	32.0	na	na	54%
4.0	36.0	456	na	14.0	na	na	44%
3.0	26.0	327	na	10.0	na	na	44%
22.0	37.0	840	na	36.0	na	78	58%
28.0	34.0	744	na	29.0	na	92	50%
11.0	27.0	480	na	9.0	na	27	34%
27.0	35.0	1088	na	39.0	na	99	58%
30.0	29.0	1007	na	33.0	na	100	55%
14.0	85.0	513	na	19.0	na	27	33%
10.0	72.0	378	na	9.0	na	36	20%
13.0	60.0	325	na	10.0	na	40	24%

Food Name	Serving Size	Total Calories
POTATOES, HASH BROWN	1 serving	235
SALAD	1 serving	11

BURGER KING

APPLE PIE	1 serving	311
BACON BITS	1 pkt	16
BAGEL		
plain	1 bagel	272
w/cream cheese	1 bagel	370
BARBECUE SAUCE		
....	1 oz	36
'Bull's-Eye'	.5 oz	22
BISCUIT, plain	1 serving	332
BREAKFAST		
French toast sticks	1 serving	440
scrambled egg platter, regular	1 serving	549
scrambled egg platter, w/bacon	1 serving	610
scrambled egg platter, w/sausage	1 serving	768
BREAKFAST SANDWICH		
bagel, w/bacon, egg, and cheese	1 serving	453
bagel, w/egg and cheese	1 serving	407
bagel, w/ham, egg, and cheese	1 serving	438
bagel, w/sausage, egg, and cheese ..	1 serving	626
biscuit, w/bacon	1 serving	378
biscuit, w/bacon and egg	1 serving	467
biscuit, w/sausage	1 serving	478
biscuit, w/sausage and egg	1 serving	568
'Breakfast Buddy'	1 serving	255
'Croissan'wich' w/bacon, egg, and cheese	1 serving	353
'Croissan'wich' w/egg and cheese	1 serving	315

Prot. MGS	Carbs. GMS	Sodium MGS	Fiber GMS	Fat GMS	Sat. Fat GMS	Chol. MGS	% Fat Cal.
3.0	26.0	349	na	14.0	na	na	54%
1.0	3.0	8	na	0.0	0.0	na	0%
3.0	44.0	412	(mq)	14.0	4.0	4	41%
1.0	0.0	na	na	1.0	na	5	56%
10.0	44.0	438	(mq)	6.0	1.0	29	20%
12.0	45.0	523	(mq)	16.0	6.0	58	39%
0.0	9.0	397	na	0.0	0.0	0	0%
0.0	5.0	47	na	0.0	0.0	0	0%
5.0	42.0	754	(mq)	17.0	3.0	2	46%
4.0	60.0	490	(mq)	27.0	7.0	0	55%
17.0	44.0	893	(mq)	34.0	9.0	365	56%
21.0	44.0	1043	(mq)	39.0	11.0	373	58%
26.0	47.0	1271	(mq)	53.0	15.0	412	62%
21.0	46.0	872	(mq)	20.0	7.0	252	40%
19.0	46.0	759	(mq)	16.0	5.0	247	35%
25.0	46.0	1114	(mq)	17.0	6.0	266	35%
27.0	49.0	1137	(mq)	36.0	12.0	293	52%
8.0	42.0	867	(mq)	20.0	5.0	8	48%
14.0	43.0	1033	(mq)	27.0	7.0	213	52%
11.0	44.0	1007	(mq)	29.0	8.0	33	55%
17.0	45.0	1172	(mq)	36.0	10.0	238	57%
11.0	15.0	492	na	16.0	6.0	127	56%
16.0	19.0	780	(mq)	23.0	8.0	230	59%
13.0	19.0	607	(mq)	20.0	7.0	222	57%

Food Name	Serving Size	Total Calories
'Croissan'wich' w/ham, egg, and cheese	1 serving	351
'Croissan'wich' w/sausage, egg, and cheese	1 serving	534
CHEESE		
American	.9 oz	92
Swiss	.9 oz	82
CHEESEBURGER		
bacon, double	1 serving	515
bacon, double, 'Deluxe'	1 serving	592
barbecue bacon, double	1 serving	536
'Deluxe'	1 serving	390
double	1 serving	483
'Mushroom Swiss' double	1 serving	473
regular	1 serving	318
'Whopper' double, w/cheese	1 serving	935
'Whopper Jr.'	1 serving	380
'Whopper' w/cheese	1 serving	706
CHICKEN, 'Chicken Tenders'	6 pieces	236
CHICKEN SANDWICH		
'B.K. Broiler'	1 serving	379
regular	1 serving	685
CREAM CHEESE	1 oz	98
CROISSANT	1 serving	180
CROUTONS	.25 oz	31
DANISH		
apple cinnamon	1 serving	390
cheese	1 serving	406
cinnamon raisin	1 serving	449
FISH SANDWICH, fillet, 'Ocean Catch'	1 serving	495
FRENCH FRIES, med order	1 serving	372
HAMBURGER		
'Burger Buddies'	1 serving	349

Prot. MGS	Carbs. GMS	Sodium MGS	Fiber GMS	Fat GMS	Sat. Fat GMS	Chol. MGS	% Fat Cal.
19.0	20.0	1373	(mq)	22.0	7.0	236	56%
21.0	22.0	985	(mq)	40.0	14.0	258	67%
5.0	1.0	312	0	7.0	5.0	25	68%
6.0	1.0	352	0	6.0	4.0	20	66%
32.0	26.0	748	(mq)	31.0	14.0	105	54%
33.0	28.0	804	(mq)	39.0	16.0	111	59%
32.0	31.0	795	(mq)	31.0	14.0	105	52%
18.0	29.0	652	(mq)	23.0	8.0	56	53%
30.0	29.0	851	(mq)	27.0	13.0	100	50%
31.0	27.0	746	(mq)	27.0	12.0	95	51%
17.0	28.0	651	(mq)	15.0	7.0	48	42%
51.0	47.0	1245	(mq)	61.0	24.0	194	59%
16.0	29.0	660	na	22.0	7.0	50	52%
32.0	47.0	1177	(mq)	44.0	16.0	115	56%
16.0	14.0	541	(mq)	13.0	3.0	46	50%
24.0	31.0	764	(mq)	18.0	3.0	53	43%
26.0	56.0	1417	(mq)	40.0	8.0	82	53%
2.0	1.0	86	0	10.0	5.0	28	92%
4.0	18.0	285	(mq)	10.0	2.0	4	50%
1.0	5.0	90	na	1.0	na	na	29%
6.0	62.0	305	(mq)	13.0	3.0	19	30%
6.0	60.0	454	(mq)	16.0	5.0	7	35%
7.0	63.0	286	(mq)	18.0	4.0	15	36%
20.0	49.0	879	(mq)	25.0	4.0	57	45%
5.0	43.0	238	(mq)	20.0	5.0	0	48%
18.0	31.0	717	(mq)	17.0	7.0	52	44%

Food Name	Serving Size	Total Calories
'Deluxe'	1 serving	344
regular	1 serving	272
'Whopper'	1 serving	614
'Whopper' double	1 serving	844
'Whopper Jr.'	1 serving	330
HONEY SAUCE	1 oz	91
LETTUCE	.75 oz	3
MAYONNAISE	1 oz	194
MILKSHAKE		
chocolate	1 serving	326
chocolate, syrup added	1 serving	409
strawberry, syrup added	1 serving	394
vanilla	1 serving	334
MUFFIN		
blueberry, mini	1 serving	292
lemon poppyseed, mini	1 serving	318
MUSTARD	1 pkt	2
ONION	.25 oz	5
ONION RINGS	1 serving	339
PICKLE	.5 oz	1
POTATOES, HASH BROWN, 'Tater Tenders'	1 serving	213
RANCH SAUCE	1 oz	171
SALAD		
chef's, w/o dressing	1 serving	178
chunky chicken, w/o dressing	1 serving	142
garden, w/o dressing	1 serving	95
side salad, w/o dressing	1 serving	25
SALAD DRESSING		
blue cheese, 'Newman's Own'	1 pkt	300
French, 'Newman's Own'	1 pkt	290
Italian, reduced calorie, 'Newman's Own'	1 pkt	170
olive oil and vinegar, 'Newman's Own'	1 pkt	310

Prot. MGS	Carbs. GMS	Sodium MGS	Fiber GMS	Fat GMS	Sat. Fat GMS	Chol. MGS	% Fat Cal.
15.0	28.0	496	(mq)	19.0	6.0	43	50%
15.0	28.0	505	(mq)	11.0	4.0	37	36%
27.0	45.0	865	(mq)	36.0	12.0	90	53%
46.0	45.0	933	(mq)	53.0	19.0	169	57%
14.0	28.0	500	na	19.0	5.0	40	52%
0.0	23.0	12	na	0.0	0.0	0	0%
0.0	0.0	2	na	0.0	0.0	0	0%
0.0	2.0	142	0	21.0	4.0	16	97%
9.0	49.0	198	na	10.0	6.0	31	28%
10.0	68.0	248	na	11.0	6.0	33	24%
9.0	66.0	230	na	10.0	6.0	33	23%
9.0	51.0	213	(tr)	10.0	6.0	33	27%
4.0	37.0	244	(mq)	14.0	3.0	72	43%
5.0	33.0	253	(mq)	18.0	3.0	72	51%
0.0	0.0	34	na	0.0	0.0	0	0%
0.0	1.0	0	(mq)	0.0	0.0	0	0%
5.0	38.0	628	(mq)	19.0	5.0	0	50%
0.0	0.0	119	(mq)	0.0	0.0	0	0%
2.0	25.0	318	(mq)	12.0	3.0	0	51%
0.0	2.0	208	na	18.0	3.0	0	95%
17.0	7.0	568	(mq)	9.0	4.0	103	46%
20.0	8.0	443	(mq)	4.0	1.0	49	25%
6.0	8.0	125	(mq)	5.0	3.0	15	47%
1.0	5.0	27	(mq)	0.0	0.0	0	0%
3.0	2.0	512	0	32.0	7.0	58	96%
0.0	23.0	400	na	22.0	3.0	0	68%
0.0	3.0	762	na	18.0	3.0	0	95%
0.0	2.0	214	0	33.0	5.0	0	96%

Food Name	Serving Size	Total Calories
ranch, 'Newman's Own'	1 pkt	350
Thousand Island, 'Newman's Own'	1 pkt	290
SANDWICH SAUCE		
'B.K. Broiler'	.5 oz	90
'Burger King A.M. Express'	1 oz	84
SWEET AND SOUR SAUCE	1 oz	45
TARTAR SAUCE	1 oz	134
TOMATO	1 oz	6

CAPTAIN D'S

Food Name	Serving Size	Total Calories
BEANS		
green, seasoned	1 serving	46
white	1 serving	126
BREADSTICKS	1 stick	91
CHICKEN ENTRÉE, w/rice, green beans,		
breadstick, salad	1 serving	414
COCKTAIL SAUCE	2 tbsp	34
CRACKER	4 crackers	50
FISH DINNER		
baked, w/rice, green beans,		
breadstick, coleslaw	1 serving	659
orange roughy, w/rice, green beans,		
breadstick, salad	1 serving	537
RICE	1 serving	124
SALAD, dinner, w/o dressing	1 serving	27
SALAD DRESSING, Italian, low-calorie	2 tbsp	9
SHRIMP ENTRÉE, w/rice, green beans,		
breadstick, salad	1 serving	457
SWEET AND SOUR SAUCE	2 tbsp	52

Prot. MGS	Carbs. GMS	Sodium MGS	Fiber GMS	Fat GMS	Sat. Fat GMS	Chol. MGS	% Fat Cal.
1.0	4.0	316	na	37.0	7.0	20	95%
1.0	15.0	403	na	26.0	5.0	36	81%
0.0	0.0	95	na	10.0	1.0	7	100%
0.0	21.0	18	na	0.0	0.0	0	0%
0.0	11.0	52	na	0.0	0.0	0	0%
0.0	2.0	202	na	14.0	2.0	20	94%
0.0	1.0	3	(mq)	0.0	0.0	0	0%
2.0	5.0	752	na	2.0	na	4	39%
8.0	22.0	99	na	1.0	na	2	7%
3.0	17.0	210	na	1.0	na	0	10%
30.0	55.0	2615	na	8.0	na	71	17%
0.0	8.0	252	na	0.0	0.0	0	0%
1.0	8.0	147	na	1.0	na	3	18%
36.0	62.0	1767	na	30.0	na	54	41%
35.0	56.0	2156	na	19.0	na	39	32%
3.0	28.0	9	na	0.0	na	0	0%
1.0	3.0	67	na	1.0	na	1	33%
0.0	2.0	568	na	0.0	0.0	0	0%
56.0	34.0	2194	na	10.0	na	191	20%
0.0	13.0	5	na	0.0	0.0	0	0%

Food Name	Serving Size	Total Calories

CARL'S JR.

BREAKFAST

bacon, 2 strips, .4 oz	1 serving	50
eggs, scrambled, 2.4 oz	1 serving	120
French toast dips, w/o syrup	1 serving	480
hotcakes, w/margarine, w/o syrup	1 serving	360
sausage, 1 patty, .5 oz	1 serving	190
'Sunrise' w/bacon, 4.5 oz	1 serving	370
'Sunrise' w/sausage, 6.1 oz	1 serving	500
BROCCOLI SOUP, cream of	6.6 oz	140
BROWNIE, fudge, 4.5 oz	1 serving	597

CAKE

chocolate, 3 oz	1 serving	300
fudge moussecake	4 oz	400

CHEESE

American, .6 oz	1 slice	60
Swiss, .6 oz	1 slice	60

CHEESEBURGER

'Double Western Bacon' 11.6 oz	1 serving	1030
'Western Bacon' approx 8 oz	1 serving	730
CHEESECAKE	3.5 oz	310
CHICKEN NOODLE SOUP, 'Old Fashioned'	6.6 oz	80

CHICKEN SANDWICH

'Charbroiler BBQ' 'Lite Menu'	1 serving	310
'Charbroiler Chicken Club' 8.8 oz	1 serving	570
'Santa Fe' 7.9 oz	1 serving	530
'Teriyaki' 'Lite Menu'	1 serving	330
CHICKEN STRIPS	6 strips	260
CHOWDER, Boston clam	6.6 oz	140
CINNAMON ROLL, 4 oz	1 serving	460
COOKIE, chocolate chip, 2.5 oz	1 serving	330

Prot. MGS	Carbs. GMS	Sodium MGS	Fiber GMS	Fat GMS	Sat. Fat GMS	Chol. MGS	% Fat Cal.
3.0	0.0	200	0	4.0	3.0	8	72%
9.0	2.0	105	0	9.0	4.0	245	68%
8.0	54.0	576	(mq)	25.0	10.0	54	47%
7.0	59.0	1190	(mq)	12.0	3.0	15	30%
7.0	1.0	275	0	17.0	4.0	25	81%
17.0	32.0	750	(mq)	19.0	8.0	120	46%
22.0	31.0	990	(mq)	32.0	12.0	165	58%
7.0	14.0	845	(mq)	6.0	4.0	22	39%
8.0	88.0	295	(mq)	27.0	7.0	tr	41%
3.0	49.0	262	na	11.0	3.0	25	33%
5.0	42.0	85	na	23.0	11.0	110	52%
4.0	1.0	290	na	5.0	3.0	15	75%
4.0	1.0	220	na	4.0	3.0	15	60%
56.0	58.0	1810	na	63.0	32.0	145	55%
34.0	59.0	1490	na	39.0	20.0	90	48%
7.0	32.0	200	na	17.0	8.0	60	49%
4.0	11.0	605	(mq)	1.0	tr	14	11%
25.0	34.0	680	na	6.0	2.0	30	17%
35.0	42.0	1160	na	29.0	8.0	60	46%
30.0	36.0	1230	na	29.0	7.0	85	49%
28.0	42.0	830	na	6.0	2.0	55	16%
19.0	11.0	600	na	19.0	5.0	25	66%
6.0	12.0	861	(mq)	8.0	3.0	22	51%
7.0	70.0	230	na	18.0	1.0	0	35%
4.0	41.0	170	na	17.0	7.0	5	46%

Food Name	Serving Size	Total Calories
DANISH		
all varieties, except cheese	1 serving	520
cheese	4 oz	520
ENGLISH MUFFIN, w/margarine, 2 oz	1 muffin	180
FISH SANDWICH		
'Carl's Catch'	1 serving	560
fillet, 7.9 oz	1 serving	550
FRENCH FRIES		
'CrissCut' regular, approx 3.2 oz	1 serving	330
regular	1 serving	420
HAMBURGER		
'Carl's Original' 6.8 oz	1 serving	460
'Famous Star' 8.6 oz	1 serving	610
'Happy Star' 3 oz	1 serving	220
'Old Time Star' 5.9 oz	1 serving	400
regular, 4.3 oz	1 serving	320
'Super Star' 11.25 oz	1 serving	820
ICED TEA, regular size	20 oz	2
MILK, 1% lowfat	10 oz	150
MILKSHAKE, regular	11.6 oz	350
MUFFIN		
blueberry, 4.2 oz	1 muffin	340
bran, 4.7 oz	1 muffin	310
ONION RINGS		
5.3-oz order	1 serving	520
3.2-oz order	1 serving	310
ORANGE JUICE, small, 8.7 oz	1 serving	90
POTATO, BAKED, 'Fiesta' 15.2 oz	1 serving	550
ROAST BEEF SANDWICH		
'California Roast Beef 'n Swiss'	1 serving	360
'Club'	1 serving	620
'Deluxe' 9.3 oz	1 serving	540

Prot. MGS	Carbs. GMS	Sodium MGS	Fiber GMS	Fat GMS	Sat. Fat GMS	Chol. MGS	% Fat Cal.
7.0	75.0	230	na	16.0	4.0	0	28%
7.0	75.0	230	na	22.0	4.0	0	38%
4.0	28.0	275	(mq)	6.0	2.0	0	30%
17.0	54.0	1220	na	30.0	4.0	5	48%
22.0	58.0	945	(mq)	26.0	11.0	90	43%
4.0	27.0	890	na	22.0	3.0	tr	60%
4.0	54.0	200	na	20.0	5.0	0	43%
25.0	46.0	810	na	20.0	9.0	50	39%
26.0	42.0	890	na	38.0	13.0	50	56%
12.0	26.0	445	(mq)	8.0	4.0	45	33%
24.0	38.0	760	(mq)	17.0	7.0	80	38%
17.0	33.0	590	na	14.0	5.0	35	39%
43.0	41.0	1210	na	53.0	24.0	105	58%
0.0	0.0	0	na	0.0	0.0	0	0%
14.0	19.0	200	na	3.0	2.0	13	18%
11.0	61.0	230	na	7.0	4.0	15	18%
5.0	61.0	300	na	9.0	1.0	45	24%
6.0	52.0	370	na	7.0	0.0	60	20%
9.0	63.0	960	na	26.0	6.0	0	45%
4.0	38.0	260	(mq)	15.0	7.0	10	44%
2.0	21.0	2	na	1.0	0.0	0	10%
25.0	60.0	1230	(mq)	23.0	9.0	40	38%
31.0	43.0	1070	(mq)	8.0	4.0	130	20%
30.0	48.0	1950	na	34.0	11.0	45	49%
28.0	46.0	1340	na	26.0	10.0	40	43%

Food Name	Serving Size	Total Calories
SALAD		
salad-to-go, chef's, 10.7 oz	1 serving	180
salad-to-go, chicken, 'Lite Menu'	1 serving	200
salad-to-go, chicken, 12 oz	1 serving	200
salad-to-go, garden, 4.8 oz	1 serving	50
salad-to-go, garden, 'Lite Menu'	1 serving	50
salad-to-go, taco, 14.3 oz	1 serving	356
SALAD DRESSING		
1000 Island	1 oz	110
blue cheese	1 oz	150
French, reduced calorie	1 oz	40
house	1 oz	110
Italian	1 oz	120
Italian, reduced calorie	1 oz	40
SALSA	1 oz	8
STEAK SANDWICH, country-fried, 7.2 oz	1 serving	610
TURKEY SANDWICH, 'Club' 9.3 oz	1 serving	530
VEGETABLE SOUP, 'Lumber Jack Mix'	6.6 oz	70
ZUCCHINI		
fried, 4.3 oz	1 serving	300
fried, 6 oz	1 serving	390

CARVEL

Food Name	Serving Size	Total Calories
ICE CREAM		
'Carvella'	1 serving	164
'Thinny-Thin'	1 serving	92
ICE CREAM CONE		
plain	1 cone	25
sugar	1 cone	45
YOGURT, FROZEN		
'Lo-Yo'	1 serving	124
sugar-free, low-fat	1 serving	104

Prot. MGS	Carbs. GMS	Sodium MGS	Fiber GMS	Fat GMS	Sat. Fat GMS	Chol. MGS	% Fat Cal.
19.0	11.0	581	(mq)	7.0	3.0	63	35%
24.0	8.0	300	na	8.0	4.0	70	36%
24.0	8.0	300	na	8.0	4.0	70	36%
3.0	4.0	75	na	3.0	2.0	5	54%
3.0	4.0	75	na	3.0	2.0	5	54%
29.0	18.0	690	(mq)	19.0	6.0	99	48%
0.0	4.0	200	na	11.0	3.0	5	90%
1.0	0.0	250	na	15.0	3.0	20	90%
0.0	5.0	292	na	2.0	0.0	0	45%
1.0	2.0	170	(tr)	11.0	3.0	10	90%
0.0	1.0	210	(tr)	13.0	2.0	0	98%
0.0	5.0	290	na	2.0	0.0	0	45%
0.0	2.0	210	na	0.0	0.0	0	0%
25.0	54.0	1290	(mq)	33.0	12.0	45	49%
30.0	50.0	2890	na	23.0	6.0	60	39%
2.0	10.0	807	(mq)	3.0	tr	3	39%
5.0	33.0	480	(mq)	16.0	7.0	10	48%
7.0	38.0	1040	na	23.0	6.0	0	53%
4.0	16.0	92	na	8.0	na	61	44%
4.0	16.0	80	na	0.0	na	4	0%
1.0	5.0	25	na	0.0	0.0	na	0%
1.0	10.0	30	na	1.0	na	na	20%
4.0	20.0	76	na	4.0	na	16	29%
4.0	20.0	80	na	4.0	na	8	35%

Food Name	Serving Size	Total Calories

CHICK-FIL-A

Food Name	Serving Size	Total Calories
BROWNIE, fudge, w/nuts, 2.8 oz	1 brownie	369
CHEESECAKE		
plain, 3.2 oz	1 slice	299
w/blueberry topping, 4.3 oz	1 slice	350
w/strawberry topping, 4.3 oz	1 slice	343
CHICKEN ENTRÉE, salad plate	11.8 oz	875
CHICKEN NUGGET		
'Chick-Fil-A Nuggets' 8 pack	4 oz	287
'Chick-Fil-A Nuggets' 12 pack	6 oz	430
'Grilled 'n Lites' 2 skewers	1 serving	97
CHICKEN SANDWICH		
chargrilled	1 serving	258
chargrilled 'Deluxe' w/lettuce and tomato	1 serving	266
'Chick-Fil-A' w/bun	1 serving	426
'Chick-Fil-A' w/o bun	1 serving	219
'Chick-Fil-A Deluxe'	1 serving	368
'Chick-n-Q'	1 serving	409
salad, on wheat bread	5.7 oz	449
CHICKEN SOUP		
'Hearty Breast of Chicken' large	17.5 oz	432
'Hearty Breast of Chicken' medium	14 oz	230
'Hearty Breast of Chicken' small	1 serving	152
COLESLAW	1 cup	175
FRENCH FRIES, waffle, small order	3 oz	270
ICE CREAM, 'Ice Dream' small cup	4.5 oz	134
ICED TEA, unsweetened	9 oz	3
LEMON PIE	1 slice	329
LEMONADE, regular	10 oz	124
ORANGE JUICE	6 oz	82

Prot. MGS	Carbs. GMS	Sodium MGS	Fiber GMS	Fat GMS	Sat. Fat GMS	Chol. MGS	% Fat Cal.
5.0	45.0	213	>.5 c	19.0	na	30	46%
6.6	24.7	272	>1.0 c	19.1	na	13	57%
6.8	37.3	294	>1.0 c	19.2	na	13	49%
6.9	35.2	309	>1.0 c	19.2	na	13	50%
29.0	60.0	1839	na	63.0	na	97	65%
28.0	13.0	1326	na	15.0	na	61	47%
42.0	19.0	1989	na	23.0	na	92	48%
20.0	4.0	280	na	2.0	na	3	19%
30.0	24.0	1121	na	5.0	na	40	17%
31.0	26.0	1125	na	na	5.0	40	0%
42.0	40.0	1174	na	9.0	na	66	19%
36.0	2.0	552	na	7.0	na	42	29%
41.0	30.0	1178	na	9.0	na	66	22%
28.0	41.0	1197	na	15.0	na	10	33%
10.0	35.0	888	na	26.0	na	50	52%
52.0	36.0	1746	na	9.0	na	92	19%
27.0	19.0	890	na	5.0	na	80	20%
16.0	11.0	530	na	3.0	na	46	18%
1.0	11.0	158	na	14.0	na	13	72%
3.0	33.0	45	na	14.0	na	8	47%
4.0	19.0	51	na	5.0	na	24	34%
0.0	0.0	0	na	0.0	na	0	0%
8.0	64.0	300	na	5.0	na	7	14%
tr	32.0	tr	na	tr	na	tr	0%
1.0	20.0	2	na	tr	na	0	0%

Food Name	Serving Size	Total Calories
SALAD		
carrot-raisin	1 cup	116
chargrilled chicken garden, w/o dressing	1 serving	126
chicken, cup, 4 oz	1 serving	309
potato	1 cup	198
tossed	1 serving	21
tossed, w/blue cheese dressing	6 oz	243
tossed, w/honey French dressing	6 oz	277
tossed, w/lite Italian dressing	6 oz	43
tossed, w/lite ranch dressing	6 oz	114
tossed, w/ranch dressing	6 oz	298
tossed, w/Thousand Island dressing	6 oz	250
SALAD DRESSING, Italian, lite	3 tbsp	43

CHURCH'S FRIED CHICKEN

APPLE PIE	3.1 oz	280
BISCUIT	2.1 oz	250
CHICKEN		
breast, boneless, 2.8 oz	1 serving	200
breast, fried, 4.3 oz	1 serving	278
breast, wing, fried, 4.8 oz	1 serving	303
leg, 2.9 oz	1 serving	147
leg, boneless, 2 oz	1 serving	140
thigh, 4.2 oz	1 serving	306
thigh, boneless, 2.8 oz	1 serving	230
wing, boneless, 3.1 oz	1 serving	250
CHICKEN FILLET		
breast	1 serving	608
breast, w/cheese	1 serving	661
COLESLAW	3 oz	92

Prot. MGS	Carbs. GMS	Sodium MGS	Fiber GMS	Fat GMS	Sat. Fat GMS	Chol. MGS	% Fat Cal.
1.0	18.0	8	na	5.0	na	6	39%
20.0	8.0	567	na	2.0	na	28	14%
12.0	4.0	543	na	28.0	na	21	82%
3.0	14.0	337	na	15.0	na	6	68%
1.0	4.0	19	na	0.0	na	0	0%
3.0	6.0	475	>2.0 c	24.0	na	38	89%
1.0	21.0	396	>2.0 c	21.0	na	0	68%
1.0	7.0	856	>2.0 c	1.2	na	0	25%
1.0	13.2	292	>2.0 c	6.3	na	6	50%
1.0	6.0	387	>2.0 c	30.0	na	5	91%
1.0	12.0	396	>2.0 c	22.0	na	25	79%
1.0	7.0	856	na	1.0	na	0	21%
2.3	40.5	340	1.0	12.3	na	<5	40%
2.2	25.6	640	1.0	16.4	na	<5	59%
19.0	4.3	510	0	12.4	na	65	56%
21.0	9.0	560	na	17.0	na	na	55%
22.0	9.0	583	na	20.0	na	na	59%
13.0	5.0	286	na	9.0	na	na	55%
12.7	2.4	160	0	9.1	na	45	59%
19.0	9.0	448	na	22.0	na	na	65%
16.2	5.3	520	0	16.2	na	80	63%
18.5	7.7	540	0	16.1	na	60	58%
27.0	46.0	725	na	34.0	na	na	50%
30.0	47.0	921	na	38.0	na	na	52%
4.2	8.4	230	2.0	5.5	na	0	54%

Food Name	Serving Size	Total Calories
CORN		
on the cob	5.7 oz	190
on the cob, w/butter oil	1 ear	237
DESSERT, frozen	1 serving	180
FISH FILLET		
regular	1 serving	430
w/cheese	1 serving	483
FRENCH FRIES		
large order	1 serving	320
regular order, 2.7 oz	1 serving	210
HOT DOG		
super	1 serving	520
super, w/cheese	1 serving	580
super, w/chili	1 serving	570
w/cheese	1 serving	330
w/chili	1 serving	320
HUSHPUPPY	2 pieces	156
OKRA	2.8 oz	210
ONION RINGS	1 serving	280
POTATOES, MASHED, w/gravy	3.7 oz	90
RICE, Cajun	3.1 oz	130

COLOMBO

Food Name	Serving Size	Total Calories
YOGURT, FROZEN		
lite, nonfat	4 oz	95
low-fat	4 oz	99

DAIRY QUEEN/BRAZIER

Food Name	Serving Size	Total Calories
BANANA SPLIT	13 oz	510
BARBECUE SANDWICH, beef	4.5 oz	225
BARBECUE SAUCE	1 pkg	41

Prot. MGS	Carbs. GMS	Sodium MGS	Fiber GMS	Fat GMS	Sat. Fat GMS	Chol. MGS	% Fat Cal.
7.8	32.4	15	4.0	5.4	na	0	26%
4.0	33.0	20	na	9.0	na	na	34%
4.0	27.0	65	na	6.0	na	na	30%
20.0	45.0	675	na	18.0	na	na	38%
23.0	46.0	870	na	22.0	na	na	41%
3.0	40.0	185	na	16.0	na	na	45%
3.3	28.5	60	2.0	10.5	na	0	45%
17.0	44.0	1365	na	27.0	na	na	47%
22.0	45.0	1605	na	34.0	na	na	53%
21.0	47.0	1595	na	32.0	na	na	51%
15.0	21.0	990	na	21.0	na	na	57%
13.0	23.0	985	na	20.0	na	na	56%
3.0	23.0	110	na	6.0	na	na	35%
2.7	19.1	520	4.0	16.1	na	0	69%
4.0	31.0	140	na	16.0	na	na	51%
1.2	14.0	520	1.0	3.3	na	0	33%
1.3	15.6	260	<1.0	7.0	na	5	48%
4.0	21.0	70	na	0.0	na	0	0%
3.0	18.0	35	na	2.0	na	10	18%
9.0	93.0	250	(mq)	11.0	8.0	30	19%
12.0	34.0	700	(mq)	4.0	1.0	20	16%
0.0	9.0	130	na	0.0	na	0	0%

Food Name	Serving Size	Total Calories
BROWNIE, hot fudge, 'Brownie Delight'		
10.8 oz .... 1 serving		710
CAKE		
frozen, undecorated .... 5.8-oz slice		380
strawberry shortcake .... 1 serving		540
CHEESEBURGER		
double, 8 oz .... 1 serving		570
single, 5.5 oz .... 1 serving		365
triple .... 1 serving		820
CHICKEN NUGGET, all white meat .... 1 serving		276
CHICKEN SANDWICH		
fillet, breaded .... 6.7 oz		430
fillet, breaded, w/cheese .... 7.2 oz		480
fillet, grilled .... 6.5 oz		300
FISH SANDWICH		
fillet .... 6 oz		370
fillet, w/cheese .... 6.5 oz		420
FRENCH FRIES		
large order .... 4.5 oz		390
regular order .... 3.5 oz		300
FROZEN DESSERT. See also individual listings.		
'Blizzard' Heath, regular .... 14.3 oz		820
'Blizzard' Heath, small .... 10.3 oz		560
'Blizzard' strawberry, regular .... 13.5 oz		740
'Blizzard' strawberry, small .... 9.4 oz		500
'Breeze' Heath, regular .... 13.4 oz		680
'Breeze' Heath, small .... 9.6 oz		450
'Breeze' strawberry, regular .... 12.5 oz		590
'Breeze' strawberry, small .... 8.7 oz		400
'Buster Bar' .... 5.3 oz		450
'Chipper Sandwich' .... 1 serving		318
'Dilly Bar' .... 3 oz		210
'Double Delight' .... 1 serving		490

Prot. MGS	Carbs. GMS	Sodium MGS	Fiber GMS	Fat GMS	Sat. Fat GMS	Chol. MGS	% Fat Cal.
11.0	102.0	340	na	29.0	14.0	35	37%
6.0	50.0	210	na	18.0	8.0	20	43%
10.0	100.0	215	na	11.0	na	25	18%
37.0	31.0	1070	(mq)	34.0	18.0	120	54%
20.0	30.0	800	(mq)	18.0	9.0	60	44%
58.0	34.0	1010	na	50.0	na	140	55%
16.0	13.0	505	na	18.0	na	39	59%
24.0	37.0	760	(mq)	20.0	4.0	55	42%
27.0	38.0	980	(mq)	25.0	7.0	70	47%
25.0	33.0	800	(mq)	8.0	2.0	50	24%
16.0	39.0	630	(mq)	16.0	3.0	45	39%
19.0	40.0	850	(mq)	21.0	6.0	60	45%
5.0	52.0	200	(mq)	18.0	4.0	0	42%
4.0	40.0	160	(mq)	14.0	3.0	0	42%
16.0	114.0	410	na	36.0	17.0	60	40%
11.0	79.0	280	na	23.0	11.0	40	37%
13.0	92.0	230	na	16.0	11.0	50	19%
9.0	64.0	160	na	12.0	8.0	35	22%
15.0	113.0	360	na	21.0	6.0	15	28%
11.0	78.0	230	na	12.0	3.0	10	24%
12.0	90.0	170	na	1.0	<1.0	5	2%
9.0	63.0	115	na	<1.0	<1.0	5	0%
11.0	40.0	220	na	29.0	9.0	15	58%
5.0	56.0	170	na	7.0	na	13	20%
3.0	21.0	50	na	13.0	6.0	10	56%
9.0	69.0	150	na	20.0	na	25	37%

Food Name	Serving Size	Total Calories
'DQ Sandwich'	1 serving	140
'Float'	1 serving	410
'Freeze'	1 serving	500
'Fudge Nut Bar'	1 serving	406
'Mr. Misty' large	1 serving	340
'Mr. Misty' regular, 11.6 oz	1 serving	250
'Mr. Misty Float'	1 serving	390
'Mr. Misty Freeze'	1 serving	500
'Nutty Double Fudge'	9.7 oz	580
'Peanut Buster Parfait'	10.8 oz	710
'QC Big Scoop' chocolate	4.5 oz	310
'QC Big Scoop' vanilla	4.5 oz	300
HAMBURGER		
double, 7 oz	1 serving	460
'Homestyle Ultimate' 9.7 oz	1 serving	700
single, 5oz	1 serving	310
triple	1 serving	710
HOT DOG		
'DQ Hounder'	1 serving	480
'DQ Hounder' w/cheese	1 serving	533
'DQ Hounder' w/chili	1 serving	575
'1/4 lb Super Dog' 7 oz	1 serving	590
regular, 3.5 oz	1 serving	280
regular, w/cheese, 4 oz	1 serving	330
regular, w/chili, 4.5 oz	1 serving	320
super, w/cheese	1 serving	580
super, w/chili	1 serving	570
ICE CREAM CONE		
chocolate, 'Queen's Choice'	1 serving	326
chocolate, dipped, large	1 serving	570
chocolate, dipped, regular, 5.5 oz	1 serving	330
chocolate, large, 7.5 oz	1 serving	350
chocolate, regular, 5 oz	1 serving	230

Prot. MGS	Carbs. GMS	Sodium MGS	Fiber GMS	Fat GMS	Sat. Fat GMS	Chol. MGS	% Fat Cal.
3.0	24.0	40	na	4.0	na	5	26%
5.0	82.0	85	na	7.0	na	20	15%
9.0	89.0	180	na	12.0	na	30	22%
8.0	40.0	167	na	25.0	na	10	55%
tr	84.0	10	na	tr	na	0	0%
tr	63.0	10	na	tr	0.0	0	0%
5.0	74.0	95	na	7.0	na	20	16%
9.0	91.0	140	na	12.0	na	30	22%
10.0	85.0	170	(mq)	22.0	10.0	35	34%
16.0	94.0	410	(mq)	32.0	10.0	30	41%
5.0	40.0	100	na	14.0	10.0	35	41%
5.0	39.0	100	na	14.0	9.0	35	42%
31.0	29.0	630	(mq)	25.0	12.0	95	49%
43.0	30.0	1110	(mq)	47.0	21.0	140	60%
17.0	29.0	580	(mq)	13.0	6.0	45	38%
51.0	33.0	690	na	45.0	na	135	57%
16.0	21.0	1800	na	36.0	na	80	68%
19.0	22.0	1995	na	40.0	na	89	68%
22.0	25.0	1900	na	41.0	na	89	64%
20.0	41.0	1360	(mq)	38.0	16.0	60	58%
9.0	23.0	700	(mq)	16.0	6.0	25	51%
12.0	24.0	920	(mq)	21.0	9.0	35	57%
11.0	26.0	720	(mq)	19.0	7.0	30	53%
22.0	45.0	1605	na	34.0	na	100	53%
21.0	47.0	1595	na	32.0	na	100	51%
5.0	40.0	84	na	16.0	na	52	44%
9.0	64.0	145	na	24.0	na	30	38%
6.0	40.0	100	(mq)	16.0	8.0	20	44%
8.0	54.0	170	(mq)	11.0	8.0	30	28%
6.0	36.0	115	(mq)	7.0	5.0	20	27%

Food Name	Serving Size	Total Calories
vanilla, 'Queen's Choice'	1 serving	322
vanilla, large, 7.5 oz	1 serving	340
vanilla, regular, 5 oz	1 serving	230
vanilla, small, 3 oz	1 serving	140
LETTUCE	.5 oz	2
MALT		
chocolate, large	1 serving	1060
chocolate, regular	1 serving	760
chocolate, small	1 serving	520
'Queen' large, 21 oz	1 serving	889
vanilla, regular, 14.7 oz	1 serving	610
MILKSHAKE		
chocolate, large	1 serving	990
chocolate, regular, 14 oz	1 serving	540
chocolate, small	1 serving	490
'Queen' large, 21 oz	1 serving	831
vanilla, large, 16.3 oz	1 serving	600
vanilla, regular, 14 oz	1 serving	520
ONION RINGS	3 oz	240
SALAD		
garden, w/o dressing	10 oz	200
side order, w/o dressing	4.8 oz	25
SALAD DRESSING		
French, reduced calorie	2 oz	90
Thousand Island	2 oz	225
SUNDAE		
chocolate, large	1 serving	440
chocolate, regular, 6.2 oz	1 serving	300
strawberry, waffle cone, 6.1 oz	1 serving	350
TOMATO	.5 oz	4
YOGURT, FROZEN		
cone, large	7.5 oz	260
cone, regular	5 oz	180

Prot. MGS	Carbs. GMS	Sodium MGS	Fiber GMS	Fat GMS	Sat. Fat GMS	Chol. MGS	% Fat Cal.
4.0	40.0	71	na	16.0	na	52	45%
9.0	53.0	140	(mq)	10.0	7.0	30	26%
6.0	36.0	95	(mq)	7.0	5.0	20	27%
4.0	22.0	60	(mq)	4.0	3.0	15	26%
0.0	0.0	1	na	0.0	na	0	0%
20.0	187.0	360	na	25.0	na	70	21%
14.0	134.0	260	na	18.0	na	50	21%
10.0	91.0	180	na	13.0	na	35	23%
16.0	157.0	304	na	21.0	na	60	21%
13.0	106.0	230	na	14.0	8.0	45	21%
19.0	168.0	360	na	26.0	na	70	24%
12.0	94.0	290	na	14.0	8.0	45	23%
10.0	82.0	180	na	13.0	na	35	24%
16.0	140.0	304	na	22.0	na	60	24%
13.0	101.0	260	na	16.0	10.0	50	24%
12.0	88.0	230	na	14.0	8.0	45	24%
4.0	29.0	135	(mq)	12.0	3.0	0	45%
13.0	7.0	240	(mq)	13.0	7.0	185	59%
1.0	4.0	15	(mq)	0.0	0.0	0	0%
<1.0	11.0	450	0	5.0	1.0	0	50%
<1.0	10.0	570	0	21.0	3.0	25	84%
8.0	78.0	165	na	10.0	na	30	20%
6.0	54.0	100	na	7.0	5.0	20	21%
8.0	56.0	220	na	12.0	5.0	20	31%
0.0	1.0	10	na	0.0	na	0	0%
9.0	56.0	115	0	<1.0	<1.0	5	<4%
6.0	38.0	80	0	<1.0	<1.0	5	<5%

Food Name	Serving Size	Total Calories
cup, regular	5 oz	170
cup, large	7 oz	230
strawberry sundae, regular	12.5 oz	200

DEL TACO

Food Name	Serving Size	Total Calories
BREAKFAST BURRITO	1 burrito	256
BURRITO		
beef, 'Del'	1 serving	440
'Big Del'	1 serving	453
chicken	1 serving	264
chicken fajita, 'Deluxe'	1 serving	435
combination	1 serving	413
green	1 serving	229
green, large	1 serving	330
red	1 serving	235
red, large	1 serving	342
CHEESEBURGER	1 serving	284
FRENCH FRIES	1 serving	242
GUACAMOLE	2 tbsp	60
HAMBURGER	1 serving	231
HOT SAUCE	1 tbsp	2
MILK, 1% low-fat	1 serving	126
ORANGE JUICE	1 serving	83
REFRIED BEANS, w/cheese	1 serving	122
SALSA	4 tbsp	14
TACO		
chicken fajita, 'Deluxe'	1 serving	211
soft	1 serving	146
soft, regular	1 serving	211

Prot. MGS	Carbs. GMS	Sodium MGS	Fiber GMS	Fat GMS	Sat. Fat GMS	Chol. MGS	% Fat Cal.
6.0	35.0	70	0	<1.0	<1.0	5	<6%
8.0	49.0	100	0	<1.0	<1.0	5	<4%
6.0	43.0	80	na	<1.0	<1.0	5	<5%
9.0	30.0	409	na	11.0	na	90	39%
23.0	43.0	878	na	20.0	na	63	41%
22.0	49.0	1047	na	20.0	na	59	40%
13.0	32.0	771	na	10.0	na	36	34%
22.0	41.0	944	na	22.0	na	84	46%
21.0	46.0	1035	na	17.0	na	49	37%
9.0	32.0	714	na	8.0	na	15	31%
14.0	46.0	1149	na	11.0	na	22	30%
10.0	32.0	656	na	8.0	na	17	31%
14.0	46.0	1149	na	11.0	na	22	29%
14.0	26.0	852	na	13.0	na	42	41%
3.0	32.0	136	na	11.0	na	0	41%
1.0	2.0	130	na	6.0	na	0	90%
11.0	26.0	649	na	8.0	na	29	31%
0.0	1.0	38	0	0.0	na	0	0%
10.0	15.0	152	na	3.0	na	12	21%
1.0	20.0	19	na	0.0	na	0	0%
7.0	17.0	890	na	7.0	na	9	52%
1.0	3.0	308	na	0.0	na	1	0%
11.0	18.0	492	na	10.0	na	53	43%
5.0	17.0	223	na	6.0	na	16	37%
9.0	19.0	320	na	10.0	na	32	43%

Food Name	Serving Size	Total Calories

DENNY'S

BAGEL	1 bagel	240
BEANS, green	3 oz	13
BEEF BARLEY SOUP	1 bowl	79
BISCUIT	1 biscuit	217
BREAKFAST		
bacon	1 slice	48
egg	1 egg	80
eggs Benedict	1 serving	658
French toast	2 slices	729
ham	1 slice	156
pancake	1 pancake	136
sausage	1 link	113
waffle	1 waffle	261
CARROTS	3 oz	17
CHEESE		
American	1 slice	55
Jack	1 slice	52

D'LITES OF AMERICA

BROCCOLI SOUP, cream of	1 serving	180
CHEESE, lite	1 slice	53
CHEESEBURGER		
w/bacon, on multigrain bun	1 serving	370
w/bacon, on sesame seed bun	1 serving	370
CHICKEN SANDWICH		
fillet, on multigrain bun	1 serving	280
fillet, on sesame seed bun	1 serving	280
D'LITE SOUP	1 serving	130
DESSERT, 'Chocolate D'Lite'	1 serving	203

Prot. MGS	Carbs. GMS	Sodium MGS	Fiber GMS	Fat GMS	Sat. Fat GMS	Chol. MGS	% Fat Cal.
9.0	47.0	450	na	1.0	na	na	4%
0.8	2.6	22	na	0.1	na	na	7%
5.0	11.0	847	na	2.0	na	na	23%
4.0	35.0	800	na	7.0	na	na	29%
3.0	0.5	142	na	4.0	na	na	75%
6.0	0.0	0	na	6.0	na	na	68%
32.9	20.2	2197	na	35.6	na	na	49%
12.0	46.0	275	na	56.0	na	na	69%
14.0	1.0	1303	na	7.0	na	na	40%
4.0	26.0	656	na	2.0	na	na	13%
2.5	0.0	250	na	10.0	na	na	80%
6.0	35.0	62	na	10.0	na	na	34%
0.4	3.8	31	na	0.0	na	na	0%
3.0	0.5	230	na	1.5	na	na	25%
5.5	0.2	195	na	4.3	na	na	74%
8.0	21.0	na	na	7.0	na	na	35%
5.0	2.0	na	na	3.0	na	na	51%
32.0	20.0	na	na	18.0	na	na	44%
32.0	20.0	na	na	18.0	na	na	44%
23.0	24.0	na	na	11.0	na	na	35%
23.0	24.0	na	na	11.0	na	na	35%
14.0	10.0	na	na	4.0	na	na	28%
6.0	36.0	na	na	4.0	na	na	18%

Food Name	Serving Size	Total Calories
FISH SANDWICH		
fillet, on multigrain bun	1 serving	390
fillet, on sesame bun	1 serving	390
FRENCH FRIES		
large order	1 serving	320
regular order	1 serving	260
HAM AND CHEESE SANDWICH		
on multigrain bun	1 serving	280
on sesame seed bun	1 serving	280
HAMBURGER		
'Double D'Lite' on multigrain bun	1 serving	450
'Double D'Lite' on sesame seed bun	1 serving	450
'Jr. D'Lite' on multigrain bun	1 serving	200
'Jr. D'Lite' on sesame seed bun	1 serving	200
'1/4 lb D'Lite' on multigrain bun	1 serving	280
'1/4 lb D'Lite' on sesame seed bun	1 serving	280
POTATO, BAKED		
'Mexican'	1 serving	510
regular	1 serving	230
w/bacon and cheddar cheese	1 serving	490
w/broccoli and cheddar cheese	1 serving	410
POTATO SKINS		
'Mexi Skins'	1 piece	99
regular	1 piece	90
SALAD BAR PLATTER	1 serving	130
SALAD DRESSING, mayonnaise, lite	1 tbsp	40
TARTAR SAUCE, lite	1 tbsp	60
VEGETARIAN SANDWICH,		
'Vegetarian D'Lite'	1 serving	270

DUNKIN' DONUTS

CORN MUFFIN, 3.4 oz	1 muffin	340

Prot. MGS	Carbs. GMS	Sodium MGS	Fiber GMS	Fat GMS	Sat. Fat GMS	Chol. MGS	% Fat Cal.
22.0	29.0	na	na	21.0	na	na	48%
22.0	29.0	na	na	21.0	na	na	48%
4.0	42.0	na	na	15.0	na	na	42%
3.0	34.0	na	na	12.0	na	na	42%
27.0	26.0	na	na	8.0	na	na	26%
27.0	26.0	na	na	8.0	na	na	26%
44.0	19.0	na	na	22.0	na	na	44%
44.0	19.0	na	na	22.0	na	na	44%
15.0	19.0	na	na	7.0	na	na	32%
15.0	19.0	na	na	7.0	na	na	32%
25.0	19.0	na	na	12.0	na	na	39%
25.0	19.0	na	na	12.0	na	na	39%
27.0	61.0	na	na	18.0	na	na	32%
6.0	50.0	na	na	1.0	na	na	4%
25.0	52.0	na	na	20.0	na	na	37%
15.0	51.0	na	na	16.0	na	na	35%
4.0	6.0	na	na	7.0	na	na	64%
3.0	6.0	na	na	6.0	na	na	60%
10.0	9.0	na	na	6.0	na	na	42%
tr	1.0	na	na	4.0	na	na	90%
tr	2.0	na	na	6.0	na	na	90%
16.0	20.0	na	na	14.0	na	na	47%
7.0	51.0	560	na	12.0	na	40	32%

Food Name	Serving Size	Total Calories
CROISSANT		
almond, 3.7 oz	1 croissant	420
chocolate, 3.3 oz	1 croissant	440
plain, 2.5 oz	1 croissant	310
DONUT		
apple filled, w/cinnamon sugar, 2.8 oz	1 donut	250
Bavarian, filled w/chocolate	1 donut	240
blueberry filled, 2.4 oz	1 donut	210
'Boston Kreme'	1 donut	240
buttermilk, glazed, 2.6 oz	1 donut	290
chocolate, glazed, 2.5 oz	1 donut	324
cinnamon, apple filled	1 donut	190
coffee roll, glazed, 2.9 oz	1 donut	280
cruller, honey dipped	1 donut	260
French cruller, w/glaze, 1.3 oz	1 donut	140
jelly filled, 2.4 oz	1 donut	220
lemon filled, 2.8 oz	1 donut	260
plain, cake, 2.2 oz	1 donut	270
plain, cake, w/handle	1 donut	240
powdered, cake	1 donut	270
whole wheat, glazed, 2.9 oz	1 donut	330
yeast, chocolate frosted, 1.9 oz	1 donut	200
yeast, glazed, 1.9 oz	1 donut	200
yeast, honey dipped	1 donut	200
MUFFIN		
apple and spice, 3.5 oz	1 muffin	300
banana nut, 3.6 oz	1 muffin	310
blueberry, 3.6 oz	1 muffin	280
bran, w/raisins, 3.7 oz	1 muffin	310
cranberry nut	1 muffin	290
oat bran, plain, 3.4 oz	1 muffin	330

Prot. MGS	Carbs. GMS	Sodium MGS	Fiber GMS	Fat GMS	Sat. Fat GMS	Chol. MGS	% Fat Cal.
8.0	38.0	280	3.0	27.0	(mq)	0	58%
7.0	38.0	220	3.0	29.0	(mq)	0	59%
7.0	27.0	240	2.0	19.0	(mq)	0	55%
5.0	33.0	280	1.0	11.0	(mq)	0	40%
5.0	32.0	260	2.0	11.0	(mq)	0	41%
4.0	29.0	240	2.0	8.0	(mq)	0	34%
4.0	30.0	250	na	11.0	2.0	0	41%
4.0	37.0	370	1.0	14.0	(mq)	10	43%
3.5	34.0	383	1.9	21.0	(mq)	2	58%
4.0	25.0	220	na	9.0	2.0	0	43%
5.0	37.0	310	2.0	12.0	(mq)	0	39%
4.0	36.0	330	na	11.0	2.0	0	38%
2.0	16.0	130	0	8.0	(mq)	30	51%
4.0	31.0	230	1.0	9.0	(mq)	0	37%
4.0	33.0	280	1.0	12.0	(mq)	0	42%
4.0	25.0	330	1.0	17.0	(mq)	10	57%
4.0	26.0	370	na	14.0	3.0	0	53%
3.0	28.0	340	na	16.0	3.0	0	53%
4.0	39.0	380	2.0	18.0	(mq)	5	49%
4.0	25.0	190	1.0	10.0	(mq)	0	45%
4.0	26.0	230	1.0	9.0	(mq)	0	41%
4.0	26.0	230	na	9.0	2.0	0	41%
6.0	52.0	360	2.0	8.0	(mq)	25	24%
7.0	49.0	410	3.0	10.0	(mq)	30	29%
6.0	46.0	340	na	8.0	na	30	26%
6.0	51.0	560	4.0	9.0	(mq)	15	26%
6.0	44.0	360	na	9.0	na	25	28%
7.0	50.0	450	na	11.0	na	0	30%

Food Name	Serving Size	Total Calories

EL POLLO LOCO

BEANS, 4 oz	1 serving	100
BURRITO		
bean, rice, cheese	9 oz	530
chicken	7 oz	310
chicken, 'Classic'	9.5 oz	560
chicken, 'Loco Grande'	13.2 oz	680
chicken, spicy hot	10 oz	570
chicken, whole wheat	10.5 oz	510
steak	6 oz	450
steak, grilled	11 oz	740
vegetarian	6 oz	340
CHEESE, cheddar	1 oz	90
CHEESECAKE	3.5 oz	310
CHICKEN		
breast	3 oz	160
leg	1.75 oz	90
thigh	2 oz	180
wing	1.5 oz	110
COLESLAW	3 oz	90
CORN	3 oz	110
DESSERT		
'Orange Bang'	7 oz	110
'Pina Colada Bang'	7 oz	110
FAJITA MEAL		
chicken, w/rice, beans, 3 tortillas, salsa	17.5 oz	780
steak	17.5 oz	1040
GUACAMOLE	1 oz	60
MUSTARD, honey Dijon	1 oz	50
PASTRY, churro	1.5 oz	140
RICE	2 oz	110

Prot. MGS	Carbs. GMS	Sodium MGS	Fiber GMS	Fat GMS	Sat. Fat GMS	Chol. MGS	% Fat Cal.
5.0	16.0	460	8.0	2.5	0.5	0	23%
18.0	86.0	730	na	13.0	5.0	15	22%
23.0	30.0	510	4.0	11.0	2.0	65	32%
31.0	66.0	1170	na	20.0	8.0	75	32%
34.0	70.0	1290	na	30.0	12.0	90	40%
31.0	66.0	1180	na	20.0	8.0	75	32%
25.0	67.0	900	na	16.0	5.0	60	28%
31.0	31.0	740	4.0	22.0	9.0	70	44%
40.0	81.0	1180	na	29.0	13.0	75	35%
14.0	54.0	360	7.0	7.0	2.0	20	19%
7.0	3.0	180	0	5.0	3.0	27	50%
8.0	30.0	230	0	18.0	9.0	60	52%
26.0	0.0	390	0	6.0	2.0	110	34%
11.0	0.0	150	0	5.0	1.5	75	50%
16.0	0.0	230	0	12.0	4.0	130	60%
12.0	0.0	220	0	6.0	2.0	80	49%
1.0	7.0	35	1.0	8.0	0.0	0	80%
3.0	20.0	110	1.0	2.0	1.0	0	16%
0.0	26.0	24	0	0.0	0.0	0	0%
0.0	26.0	24	0	0.0	0.0	0	0%
41.0	120.0	1060	17.0	18.0	3.0	58	21%
61.0	120.0	1550	17.0	38.0	14.0	100	33%
1.0	2.0	130	0	6.0	0.0	0	90%
1.0	7.0	440	0	0.5	0.0	0	9%
2.0	4.0	180	0	9.0	1.8	4	58%
1.0	19.0	220	0	1.5	0.0	0	12%

Food Name	Serving Size	Total Calories
SALAD		
chicken, flame-broiled	12 oz	160
potato	4 oz	180
side order	9 oz	50
SALAD DRESSING		
blue cheese	1 oz	80
French, 'Deluxe'	1 oz	60
Italian, reduced calorie	1 oz	25
ranch	1 oz	75
Thousand Island	1 oz	110
SALSA	2 oz	10
SOUR CREAM	1 oz	60
TACO		
chicken	5 oz	180
steak	4.5 oz	250
TORTILLA		
corn	1 tortilla	60
flour	1 tortilla	90

EVERYTHING YOGURT

YOGURT, FROZEN		
low-fat	1 serving	95
nonfat	1 serving	80

GODFATHER'S PIZZA

PIZZA		
Cheese		
golden crust, large	1/10 pie	261
golden crust, medium	1/8 pie	229
golden crust, small	1/6 pie	213
original crust, large	1/10 pie	271

Prot. MGS	Carbs. GMS	Sodium MGS	Fiber GMS	Fat GMS	Sat. Fat GMS	Chol. MGS	% Fat Cal.
22.0	11.0	440	4.0	4.0	1.0	45	23%
2.0	21.0	340	1.0	10.0	1.5	10	50%
3.0	10.0	30	4.0	1.0	0.0	0	18%
1.0	4.0	150	0	6.0	1.0	5	68%
<1.0	7.0	160	0	4.0	0.0	0	60%
0.0	2.0	170	0	2.0	0.0	0	72%
<1.0	4.0	190	0	6.0	0.0	0	72%
<1.0	4.0	240	0	10.0	0.0	5	82%
1.0	3.0	180	1.0	0.0	0.0	0	0%
1.0	1.0	15	0	6.0	4.0	13	90%
13.0	18.0	300	2.0	7.0	1.0	35	35%
18.0	18.0	410	2.0	12.0	4.0	40	43%
1.0	13.0	25	<1.0	0.5	0.0	0	8%
3.0	15.0	150	<1.0	2.5	1.5	0	25%
3.0	18.0	30	na	1.0	na	5	9%
3.0	17.0	40	na	0.0	0.0	0	0%
8.0	31.0	314	na	11.0	na	23	38%
8.0	28.0	272	na	9.0	na	19	35%
8.0	27.0	258	na	8.0	na	19	34%
12.0	37.0	329	na	8.0	na	28	27%

Food Name	Serving Size	Total Calories
original crust, medium	1/8 pie	242
original crust, mini	1/4 pie	138
original crust, small	1/6 pie	239
thin crust, large	1/10 pie	228
thin crust, medium	1/8 pie	210
thin crust, small	1/6 pie	180
Combo		
golden crust, large	1/10 pie	322
golden crust, medium	1/8 pie	283
golden crust, small	1/6 pie	273
original crust, large	1/10 pie	332
original crust, medium	1/8 pie	318
original crust, mini	1/4 pie	164
original crust, small	1/6 pie	299
thin crust, large	1/10 pie	336
thin crust, medium	1/8 pie	310
thin crust, small	1/6 pie	270
PIZZA, STUFFED		
cheese, large	1/10 pie	381
cheese, medium	1/8 pie	350
cheese, small	1/6 pie	310
combo, large	1/10 pie	521
combo, medium	1/8 pie	480
combo, small	1/6 pie	430

GOLDEN CORRAL

BREAD, 'Texas Toast'	1 serving	170
CHICKEN, 'Golden Grilled'	1 serving	170
CHICKEN FILLET, 'Golden Fried'	1 serving	370
POTATO, BAKED	1 serving	220
RIBEYE STEAK, regular, 5.11 oz	1 serving	450
SHRIMP, 'Golden Fried'	1 serving	250

Prot. MGS	Carbs. GMS	Sodium MGS	Fiber GMS	Fat GMS	Sat. Fat GMS	Chol. MGS	% Fat Cal.
10.0	35.0	285	na	7.0	na	22	26%
6.0	20.0	159	na	4.0	na	13	26%
10.0	32.0	289	na	7.0	na	25	26%
11.0	28.0	464	(mq)	7.0	(mq)	16	28%
10.0	26.0	410	(mq)	7.0	(mq)	14	30%
9.0	21.0	370	(mq)	6.0	(mq)	10	30%
14.0	33.0	602	na	15.0	na	34	42%
13.0	30.0	526	na	13.0	na	29	41%
13.0	29.0	542	na	12.0	na	31	40%
16.0	39.0	617	na	12.0	na	39	33%
16.0	37.0	569	na	12.0	na	38	34%
8.0	21.0	287	na	5.0	na	17	27%
15.0	34.0	573	na	11.0	na	37	33%
17.0	31.0	870	(mq)	16.0	(mq)	27	43%
15.0	29.0	790	(mq)	14.0	(mq)	25	41%
13.0	23.0	710	(mq)	13.0	(mq)	25	43%
16.0	44.0	677	(mq)	16.0	(mq)	32	38%
14.0	42.0	610	(mq)	13.0	(mq)	25	33%
13.0	38.0	560	(mq)	11.0	(mq)	25	32%
23.0	47.0	1204	(mq)	26.0	(mq)	48	45%
21.0	45.0	1105	(mq)	23.0	(mq)	43	43%
19.0	41.0	1000	(mq)	20.0	(mq)	40	42%
5.0	26.0	230	na	6.0	na	0	32%
32.0	0.0	520	na	5.0	na	100	26%
37.0	14.0	570	na	19.0	na	85	46%
5.0	46.0	60	na	2.0	na	0	8%
34.0	0.0	220	na	35.0	na	120	70%
12.0	24.0	470	na	12.0	na	90	43%

Food Name	Serving Size	Total Calories
SIRLOIN STEAK	5 oz	230
STEAK ENTRÉE		
chopped sirloin, approx 4 oz	1 serving	320
sirloin tips, w/onions and pepper,		
approx 8.2 oz	1 serving	290

HARDEE'S

Food Name	Serving Size	Total Calories
APPLE TURNOVER	3.2 oz	270
BARBECUE SAUCE		
dipping sauce	.5-oz pkt	14
dipping sauce	1 oz	30
BISCUIT		
'Canadian Rise 'N Shine' 5.8 oz	1 serving	570
'Cinnamon 'N Raisin' 2.8 oz	1 serving	370
'Rise 'N Shine'	1 serving	390
BREAKFAST		
'Big Country Breakfast' bacon	1 serving	740
'Big Country Breakfast' ham, 8.9 oz . . .	1 serving	620
'Big Country Breakfast' sausage	1 serving	930
'Biscuit 'N Gravy' 7.8 oz	1 serving	510
biscuit, bacon, egg, and cheese	1 serving	530
biscuit, bacon, 3.3 oz	1 serving	360
biscuit, bacon and egg, 4.4 oz	1 serving	490
biscuit, chicken	1 serving	510
biscuit, country ham	1 serving	430
biscuit, country ham and egg, 4.9 oz . .	1 serving	400
biscuit, ham	1 serving	400
biscuit, ham, egg, and cheese	1 serving	500
biscuit, ham and egg, 4.9 oz	1 serving	370
biscuit, sausage, 4.2 oz	1 serving	510
biscuit, sausage and egg, 5.3 oz	1 serving	560
biscuit, steak	1 serving	580

Prot. MGS	Carbs. GMS	Sodium MGS	Fiber GMS	Fat GMS	Sat. Fat GMS	Chol. MGS	% Fat Cal.
27.0	0.0	270	na	14.0	na	85	55%
28.0	0.0	160	na	23.0	na	100	65%
30.0	8.0	260	na	13.0	na	120	40%
3.0	38.0	250	(mq)	12.0	4.0	0	40%
0.0	4.0	140	0	0.0	0.0	0	0%
0.0	8.0	300	0	0.0	0.0	0	0%
24.0	46.0	1860	na	32.0	11.0	175	51%
3.0	48.0	450	na	18.0	5.0	0	44%
6.0	44.0	1000	na	21.0	6.0	0	48%
25.0	61.0	1800	na	43.0	13.0	305	52%
28.0	51.0	1780	(mq)	33.0	7.0	325	48%
33.0	61.0	2240	na	61.0	19.0	340	59%
10.0	55.0	1500	na	28.0	9.0	15	49%
18.0	45.0	1470	na	31.0	11.0	155	53%
10.0	34.0	950	(mq)	21.0	4.0	10	53%
15.0	44.0	1250	na	27.0	9.0	155	50%
18.0	52.0	1580	na	25.0	7.0	45	44%
15.0	45.0	1930	na	22.0	6.0	25	46%
16.0	35.0	1600	(mq)	22.0	4.0	175	50%
9.0	47.0	1340	na	20.0	6.0	15	45%
16.0	48.0	1620	na	27.0	10.0	170	49%
15.0	35.0	1050	(mq)	19.0	4.0	160	46%
14.0	44.0	1360	na	31.0	10.0	25	55%
18.0	44.0	1400	na	35.0	11.0	170	56%
15.0	56.0	1580	na	32.0	10.0	30	50%

Food Name	Serving Size	Total Calories
biscuit, steak and egg	1 serving	550
pancakes, 3 cakes	1 serving	280
pancakes, 3 cakes, w/1 sausage patty	1 serving	430
pancakes, 3 cakes, w/2 bacon strips	1 serving	350
BREAKFAST SANDWICH		
'Frisco Breakfast Sandwich' ham	1 serving	460
'Frisco Breakfast Sandwich' w/hash browns	1 serving	230
CATSUP	.5 oz	14
CHEESEBURGER		
bacon	1 serving	580
'Mushroom 'N Swiss'	1 serving	500
quarter pound	1 serving	470
regular	1 serving	300
CHICKEN, FRIED		
breast, 5.2 oz	1 serving	370
leg, 2.4 oz	1 serving	170
'Stix'	6 pieces	210
'Stix'	9 pieces	310
thigh, 4.3 oz	1 serving	330
wing, 2.3 oz	1 serving	200
CHICKEN SANDWICH		
breast, grilled, 6.8 oz	1 serving	310
'Chicken Fillet' 6.1 oz	1 serving	370
fillet	1 serving	380
grilled, 'Frisco'	1 serving	620
COLESLAW		
12-oz size	1 serving	710
4-oz size	1 serving	240
COOKIE, 'Big Cookie'	2 oz	280
FISH SANDWICH, 'Fisherman's Fillet' 7.5 oz	1 serving	480

Prot. MGS	Carbs. GMS	Sodium MGS	Fiber GMS	Fat GMS	Sat. Fat GMS	Chol. MGS	% Fat Cal.
22.0	47.0	1370	na	32.0	8.0	175	52%
8.0	56.0	890	na	2.0	1.0	15	6%
16.0	56.0	1290	na	16.0	6.0	40	33%
13.0	56.0	1130	na	9.0	3.0	25	23%
20.0	46.0	1320	na	22.0	8.0	175	43%
3.0	24.0	560	na	14.0	3.0	0	55%
<1.0	3.0	135	(tr)	<1.0	<1.0	0	0%
33.0	33.0	980	na	35.0	15.0	50	54%
31.0	35.0	1020	na	26.0	13.0	45	47%
28.0	35.0	890	na	28.0	12.0	35	54%
13.0	34.0	690	na	13.0	7.0	25	39%
29.0	29.0	1190	na	15.0	4.0	75	36%
13.0	15.0	570	na	7.0	2.0	45	37%
19.0	13.0	680	na	9.0	2.0	35	39%
28.0	20.0	1020	(mq)	14.0	3.0	55	41%
19.0	30.0	1000	na	15.0	4.0	60	41%
10.0	23.0	740	na	8.0	2.0	30	36%
24.0	34.0	890	(mq)	9.0	1.0	60	26%
19.0	44.0	1060	(mq)	13.0	2.0	55	32%
20.0	46.0	1130	na	13.0	3.0	55	31%
35.0	44.0	1730	na	34.0	10.0	95	49%
5.0	38.0	1020	na	60.0	10.0	35	76%
2.0	13.0	340	na	20.0	3.0	10	75%
4.0	41.0	150	na	12.0	4.0	15	39%
25.0	49.0	1200	na	22.0	6.0	60	41%

Food Name	Serving Size	Total Calories
FRENCH FRIES		
big, 5.5 oz	1 serving	500
'Crispy Curls' 3 oz	1 serving	300
large order, 6.1 oz	1 serving	430
medium order, 5 oz	1 serving	350
small order, 3.3 oz	1 serving	240
GRAVY		
5-oz serving	1 serving	60
1.5-oz serving	1 serving	20
HAM AND CHEESE SANDWICH,		
'Hot Ham 'N' Cheese'	1 serving	530
HAMBURGER		
'Big Deluxe'	1 serving	510
'Big Twin' 6.1 oz	1 serving	450
'Frisco'	1 serving	760
regular	1 serving	260
HONEY SAUCE	.5 oz	45
HORSERADISH	.25-oz pkt	25
HOT DOG		
all beef, 4.2 oz	1 serving	300
6.8 oz	1 serving	450
ICE CREAM CONE		
chocolate, 'Cool Twist'	4.2 oz	180
vanilla, 'Cool Twist'	4.2 oz	180
vanilla/chocolate, 'Cool Twist'	4.2 oz	170
MARGARINE-BUTTER BLEND, .2 oz	1 serving	35
MAYONNAISE	.5 oz	50
MILKSHAKE		
chocolate	11.5 oz	390
peach	13.3 oz	530
strawberry	12 oz	390
vanilla	11.5 oz	370

Prot. MGS	Carbs. GMS	Sodium MGS	Fiber GMS	Fat GMS	Sat. Fat GMS	Chol. MGS	% Fat Cal.
6.0	66.0	180	(mq)	23.0	5.0	0	41%
4.0	36.0	840	na	16.0	3.0	0	48%
6.0	59.0	190	na	18.0	5.0	0	38%
5.0	49.0	150	na	15.0	4.0	0	39%
4.0	33.0	100	na	10.0	3.0	0	38%
3.0	11.0	850	na	1.0	<1.0	5	15%
1.0	3.0	260	na	<1.0	<1.0	2	15%
18.0	49.0	1710	na	30.0	9.0	65	51%
28.0	35.0	820	na	29.0	12.0	40	51%
23.0	34.0	580	(mq)	25.0	11.0	55	50%
36.0	43.0	1280	na	50.0	18.0	70	59%
11.0	33.0	460	na	9.0	4.0	20	31%
<1.0	11.0	0	0	<1.0	<1.0	0	<3%
<1.0	1.0	35	na	2.0	<1.0	5	72%
11.0	25.0	710	(mq)	17.0	8.0	25	51%
17.0	52.0	1090	na	20.0	6.0	35	40%
4.0	29.0	85	na	4.0	3.0	15	20%
5.0	29.0	80	na	4.0	3.0	15	20%
5.0	29.0	85	na	4.0	3.0	15	21%
0.0	0.0	40	0	4.0	<1.0	5	100%
<1.0	1.0	75	0	5.0	1.0	5	90%
15.0	61.0	220	na	10.0	6.0	30	23%
12.0	95.0	220	na	11.0	7.0	45	19%
13.0	65.0	200	na	8.0	5.0	30	18%
14.0	59.0	210	na	9.0	6.0	25	22%

Food Name	Serving Size	Total Calories
MUFFIN		
blueberry	1 muffin	400
oat bran raisin	1 muffin	410
MUSTARD	.3-oz pkt	6
MUSTARD SAUCE, sweet, dipping sauce	1 oz	50
ORANGE JUICE		
11-oz size	1 serving	140
6-oz size	1 serving	83
POTATOES, HASH BROWN,		
'Hash Rounds' 2.8 oz	1 serving	230
POTATOES, MASHED		
4-oz size	1 serving	70
12-oz size	1 serving	220
ROAST BEEF SANDWICH		
'Big Roast Beef'	1 serving	350
regular	1 serving	270
SALAD		
chef's, 9.5 oz	1 serving	200
chicken, grilled, 9.8 oz	1 serving	120
chicken and pasta	14.6 oz	230
garden, 9.3 oz	1 serving	190
side order, 5 oz	1 serving	20
SALAD DRESSING		
blue cheese	2 oz	210
French, reduced calorie	2 oz	130
house	2 oz	290
Italian, reduced calorie	2 oz	90
Thousand Island	2 oz	250
SAUCE		
'Big Twin'	.5 oz	50
sweet and sour, dipping sauce	1 oz	40
SUNDAE		
caramel, 'Cool Twist'	6 oz	330

Prot. MGS	Carbs. GMS	Sodium MGS	Fiber GMS	Fat GMS	Sat. Fat GMS	Chol. MGS	% Fat Cal.
7.0	56.0	310	na	17.0	4.0	65	38%
8.0	59.0	380	na	16.0	3.0	50	35%
<1.0	<1.0	120	(tr)	<1.0	<1.0	0	0%
<1.0	10.0	160	(tr)	<1.0	<1.0	0	<12%
2.0	34.0	5	na	tr	tr	0	0%
1.0	20.0	5	na	tr	tr	0	0%
3.0	24.0	560	(mq)	14.0	3.0	0	55%
2.0	14.0	260	na	<1.0	na	0	<9%
6.0	48.0	760	na	<1.0	0.0	0	<9%
22.0	33.0	1080	na	15.0	6.0	40	39%
15.0	28.0	780	na	11.0	5.0	25	37%
20.0	5.0	910	na	13.0	8.0	45	59%
18.0	2.0	520	na	4.0	1.0	60	30%
27.0	23.0	380	(mq)	3.0	1.0	55	12%
3.0	3.0	280	na	14.0	9.0	40	66%
1.0	3.0	20	na	tr	tr	0	0%
1.0	10.0	790	0	18.0	3.0	20	77%
1.0	21.0	480	0	5.0	1.0	0	35%
1.0	6.0	510	na	29.0	4.0	25	90%
<1.0	5.0	310	(tr)	8.0	1.0	0	80%
1.0	9.0	540	na	23.0	3.0	35	83%
<1.0	4.0	35	na	4.0	<1.0	5	72%
<1.0	10.0	95	0	<1.0	<1.0	0	0%
6.0	54.0	290	(tr)	10.0	5.0	20	27%

Food Name	Serving Size	Total Calories
hot fudge, 'Cool Twist'	6 oz	320
strawberry, 'Cool Twist'	5.9 oz	260
SYRUP, pancake	1.5 oz	120
TARTAR SAUCE	.7 oz	90
TURKEY SANDWICH, 'Turkey Club' 7.3 oz	1 serving	390

HARVEY'S FOODS

Food Name	Serving Size	Total Calories
APPLE JUICE	1 serving	80
APPLE TURNOVER	1 serving	179
BREAKFAST		
pancakes	1 serving	89
sausage	1 serving	167
CHEESEBURGER	1 serving	415
CHICKEN FINGERS	1 serving	240
CHICKEN SANDWICH	1 serving	419
FRENCH FRIES	1 serving	478
HAMBURGER		
'Double'	1 serving	530
regular	1 serving	355
'Super'	1 serving	477
HOT DOG	1 serving	332
MILKSHAKE		
chocolate	1 serving	321
strawberry	1 serving	303
vanilla	1 serving	305
MUFFIN		
blueberry	1 muffin	254
bran	1 muffin	301
ONION RINGS	1 serving	288
ORANGE JUICE	1 serving	77
POTATOES, HASH BROWN	1 serving	146

Prot. MGS	Carbs. GMS	Sodium MGS	Fiber GMS	Fat GMS	Sat. Fat GMS	Chol. MGS	% Fat Cal.
8.0	50.0	260	na	10.0	5.0	25	28%
6.0	48.0	100	na	6.0	3.0	15	21%
<1.0	31.0	25	0	<1.0	1.0	0	0%
<1.0	2.0	160	na	9.0	1.0	10	90%
29.0	32.0	1280	(mq)	16.0	4.0	70	37%
2.0	20.0	na	na	2.0	na	tr	23%
1.0	28.0	na	na	7.0	na	7	35%
2.0	17.0	na	na	1.0	na	8	10%
9.0	3.0	na	na	14.0	na	12	75%
22.0	41.0	na	na	18.0	na	30	39%
15.0	18.0	na	na	12.0	na	57	45%
19.0	46.0	na	na	16.0	na	110	34%
10.0	56.0	na	na	24.0	na	5	45%
31.0	44.0	na	na	26.0	na	34	44%
18.0	40.0	na	na	14.0	na	17	35%
37.0	38.0	na	na	19.0	na	112	36%
12.0	32.0	na	na	15.0	na	50	41%
12.0	74.0	na	na	11.0	na	36	31%
11.0	69.0	na	na	10.0	na	36	30%
11.0	69.0	na	na	10.0	na	36	30%
4.0	45.0	na	na	6.0	na	tr	21%
5.0	42.0	na	na	13.0	na	tr	39%
4.0	36.0	na	na	14.0	na	5	44%
1.0	18.0	na	na	1.0	na	tr	12%
2.0	15.0	tr	na	9.0	na	2	55%

Food Name	Serving Size	Total Calories
SANDWICH, 'Western' .... 1 sandwich		347
TOAST, plain .... 1 serving		250

HUNGRY HUNTER

CHICKEN TERIYAKI, breast, boneless, charbroiled .... 1 serving		413
CRAB		
Alaskan king, w/1 tbsp butter .... 1 serving		432
Alaskan king, w/o butter .... 1 serving		332
FILET MIGNON SANDWICH, midwestern, USDA choice .... 8 oz		539
LOBSTER		
w/1 tbsp butter .... 1 serving		241
w/o butter .... 1 serving		139
POTATO, BAKED .... 1 serving		185
RED SNAPPER, fresh, cooked in 1/2 oz butter .... 1 serving		329
RICE PILAF .... 1 serving		142

JACK-IN-THE-BOX

APPLE TURNOVER, 3.9 oz .... 1 serving		354
BARBECUE SAUCE .... 1-oz pkt		44
BEEF SANDWICH, gyro .... 1 serving		620
BEEF TERIYAKI BOWL .... 1 serving		640
BREADSTICKS, sesame, .5 oz .... 1 serving		70
BREAKFAST		
pancake platter, 8.1 oz .... 1 serving		612
scrambled egg platter, 7.5 oz ...... 1 serving		559
BREAKFAST SANDWICH		
'Breakfast Jack' 4.4 oz .... 1 serving		307
crescent, Canadian bacon, 4.7 oz .... 1 serving		452

Prot. MGS	Carbs. GMS	Sodium MGS	Fiber GMS	Fat GMS	Sat. Fat GMS	Chol. MGS	% Fat Cal.
15.0	58.0	na	na	10.0	na	265	26%
8.0	48.0	na	na	3.0	na	tr	11%
71.0	9.0	237	0	8.0	na	193	17%
73.0	0.0	3436	0	13.0	na	194	27%
73.0	0.0	3319	0	2.0	na	163	5%
69.0	0.0	150	0	27.0	na	203	45%
29.0	2.0	657	0	12.0	na	133	45%
29.0	2.0	539	0	1.0	na	102	6%
4.0	43.0	13	4.0	0.0	0.0	0	0%
47.0	0.0	262	0	15.0	na	114	41%
4.0	26.0	223	1.0	2.0	na	0	13%
3.0	40.0	479	(mq)	19.0	4.4	0	48%
1.0	11.0	300	0	<1.0	<1.0	0	0%
27.0	55.0	1310	na	32.0	12.0	65	46%
28.0	124.0	930	7.0	3.0	1.0	25	4%
2.0	12.0	110	(mq)	2.0	na	<1	26%
15.0	87.0	888	(mq)	22.0	8.6	99	32%
18.0	50.0	1060	(mq)	32.0	8.7	378	52%
18.0	30.0	871	(mq)	13.0	5.1	203	38%
19.0	25.0	851	(mq)	31.0	9.7	226	62%

Food Name	Serving Size	Total Calories
crescent, sausage, 5.5 oz	1 serving	584
crescent, supreme, 5.1 oz	1 serving	547
sausage, 5.5 oz	1 serving	584
scrambled egg pocket, 6.5 oz	1 serving	431
sourdough bread, egg, ham, and cheese, 5.2 oz	1 serving	381
CHEESEBURGER		
'Bacon Bacon Cheeseburger' 8.5 oz	1 serving	705
'Jumbo Jack' 8.5 oz	1 serving	677
double, 5.3 oz	1 serving	467
patty melt, 'Old Fashioned' 7.6 oz	1 serving	713
regular, 4 oz	1 serving	315
Swiss cheese and bacon, 6.6 oz	1 serving	678
'Ultimate' 9.9 oz	1 serving	942
CHEESECAKE, 3.5 oz	1 serving	309
CHICKEN SANDWICH		
grilled, fillet, 7.4 oz	1 serving	431
smoked chicken, cheddar, and bacon	1 serving	540
spicy crispy chicken	1 serving	560
supreme, 8.6 oz	1 serving	641
w/mushrooms, 7.8 oz	1 serving	438
CHICKEN STRIPS		
4 pieces	4 oz	285
6 pieces	6.2 oz	451
CHICKEN TERIYAKI BOWL	1 serving	580
CHICKEN WINGS		
9 pieces	11 oz	1270
6 pieces	7.3 oz	846
CHIMICHANGA		
mini, 4 pieces	7.3 oz	571
mini, 6 pieces	11 oz	856
COCKTAIL SAUCE	1 oz	32
COFFEE, small	8 oz	2

Prot. MGS	Carbs. GMS	Sodium MGS	Fiber GMS	Fat GMS	Sat. Fat GMS	Chol. MGS	% Fat Cal.
22.0	28.0	1012	(mq)	43.0	15.5	187	66%
20.0	27.0	1053	(mq)	40.0	13.2	178	66%
22.0	28.0	1012	(mq)	43.0	15.5	187	66%
29.0	31.0	1060	(mq)	21.0	7.5	354	44%
21.0	31.0	1120	(mq)	20.0	7.1	236	47%
35.0	41.0	1240	(mq)	45.0	14.9	113	57%
32.0	46.0	1090	(mq)	40.0	14.0	102	53%
21.0	33.0	842	(mq)	27.0	12.3	72	52%
33.0	42.0	1360	(mq)	46.0	14.8	92	58%
15.0	33.0	746	(mq)	14.0	5.7	41	40%
31.0	34.0	1458	(mq)	47.0	20.0	92	62%
47.0	33.0	1176	(mq)	69.0	26.4	127	66%
8.0	29.0	208	na	18.0	9.4	63	52%
29.0	36.0	1070	(mq)	19.0	4.7	65	40%
30.0	37.0	1520	9.0	30.0	11.0	80	50%
24.0	55.0	1020	na	27.0	5.0	50	43%
27.0	47.0	1470	(mq)	39.0	10.0	85	55%
28.0	40.0	1340	(mq)	18.0	4.9	61	37%
25.0	18.0	695	(mq)	13.0	3.1	52	41%
39.0	28.0	1100	(mq)	20.0	4.9	82	40%
28.0	115.0	1220	6.0	1.5	na	30	2%
51.0	117.0	2560	(mq)	66.0	16.0	272	47%
34.0	78.0	1710	(mq)	44.0	10.7	181	47%
22.0	57.0	633	(mq)	28.0	8.6	64	44%
34.0	85.0	949	(mq)	42.0	13.0	95	44%
<1.0	6.8	206	na	<1.0	<1.0	0	0%
0.0	0.0	26	0	0.0	0.0	0	0%

Food Name	Serving Size	Total Calories
DESSERT, double fudge, 3.0 oz	1 serving	288
EGG ROLL, 5 pieces	10 oz	753
FAJITA SANDWICH		
beef fajita pita, 6.2 oz	1 serving	333
chicken fajita pita, 6.7 oz	1 serving	292
FISH SANDWICH, supreme, 7.7 oz	1 serving	510
FRENCH FRIES		
curly, seasoned, 3.8 oz	1 serving	358
jumbo order, 4.3 oz	1 serving	396
regular order, 3.8 oz	1 serving	351
small order, 2.4 oz	1 serving	219
GUACAMOLE	1 oz	30
HAMBURGER		
'Jumbo Jack' 7.8 oz	1 serving	584
regular, 3.4 oz	1 serving	267
HOT SAUCE, .5 oz	1 serving	4
ICED TEA, small	16 oz	4
ITALIAN SAUCE	1.5 oz	28
JELLY, grape	.5 oz	38
MAYO-MUSTARD SAUCE	.7 oz	124
MAYO-ONION SAUCE	.7 oz	143
MILK, 2%	8.6 oz	122
MILKSHAKE		
chocolate	11.4 oz	330
strawberry	11.6 oz	320
vanilla	11.2 oz	320
ONION RINGS, 3.6 oz	1 serving	380
ORANGE JUICE	6.5 oz	80
POTATOES, HASH BROWN, 2.0 oz	1 serving	156
RAVIOLI		
toasted, 7 pieces	5.8 oz	537
toasted, 10 pieces	8.3 oz	768

Prot. MGS	Carbs. GMS	Sodium MGS	Fiber GMS	Fat GMS	Sat. Fat GMS	Chol. MGS	% Fat Cal.
4.0	49.0	259	(mq)	9.0	2.2	20	28%
5.0	92.0	1640	(mq)	41.0	11.7	49	49%
24.0	27.0	635	(mq)	14.0	5.9	45	38%
24.0	29.0	703	(mq)	8.0	2.9	34	25%
24.0	44.0	1040	(mq)	27.0	6.1	55	48%
5.0	39.0	1030	(mq)	20.0	4.7	0	50%
5.0	51.0	219	(mq)	19.0	4.5	0	43%
4.0	45.0	194	(mq)	17.0	4.0	0	44%
3.0	28.0	121	(mq)	11.0	2.5	0	45%
1.0	2.0	128	(mq)	3.0	<1.0	0	90%
26.0	42.0	733	(mq)	34.0	11.0	73	52%
13.0	28.0	556	(mq)	11.0	4.1	26	37%
<1.0	1.0	112	0	0.0	0.0	0	0%
1.0	<1.0	6	0	0.0	0.0	0	0%
<1.0	6.0	176	0	<1.0	<1.0	<1	0%
0.0	9.0	3	0	0.0	0.0	0	0%
0.5	2.0	247	0	13.0	na	10	94%
0.3	1.0	140	0	15.0	na	20	94%
8.0	12.0	122	0	5.0	2.9	18	37%
11.0	55.0	270	(tr)	7.0	4.3	25	19%
10.0	55.0	240	(tr)	7.0	4.3	25	20%
10.0	57.0	230	0	6.0	3.6	25	17%
5.0	38.0	451	(mq)	23.0	5.5	0	54%
1.0	20.0	0	0	0.0	0.0	0	0%
1.0	14.0	312	(mq)	11.0	2.6	0	63%
15.0	57.0	639	(mq)	28.0	8.0	36	47%
22.0	81.0	913	(mq)	40.0	11.4	52	47%

Food Name	Serving Size	Total Calories
SALAD		
chef's, 11.7 oz	1 serving	325
Mexican chicken, 14.6 oz	1 serving	442
side order, 4 oz	1 serving	51
taco, 14.2 oz	1 serving	503
SALAD DRESSING		
blue cheese	2.5-oz pkt	262
buttermilk, house	2.5-oz pkt	362
French, reduced calorie	2.5-oz pkt	176
Italian, low calorie	2.5-oz pkt	25
Thousand Island	2.5-oz pkt	312
SALSA	1 oz	8
SHRIMP		
15 pieces	4.4 oz	404
10 pieces	3.0 oz	270
SOFT DRINK		
Coca-Cola, small	16 oz	192
Diet Coke, small	16 oz	1
Dr. Pepper, small	16 oz	192
Ramblin' Root Beer, small	16 oz	235
Sprite, small	16 oz	192
STEAK SANDWICH		
country-fried, 5.4 oz	1 serving	450
sirloin, 8.4 oz	1 serving	517
SWEET AND SOUR SAUCE	1 oz	40
SYRUP, pancake	1.5 oz	121
TACO		
regular, 3 oz	1 serving	187
super, 4.5 oz	1 serving	281
TAQUITO		
5 pieces	5 oz	363
7 pieces	7 oz	508

Prot. MGS	Carbs. GMS	Sodium MGS	Fiber GMS	Fat GMS	Sat. Fat GMS	Chol. MGS	% Fat Cal.
30.0	10.0	900	(mq)	18.0	8.4	142	50%
28.0	30.0	1500	(mq)	23.0	8.6	89	47%
7.0	<1.0	84	(mq)	3.0	2.0	<1	53%
34.0	28.0	1600	(mq)	31.0	13.4	92	55%
<1.0	14.0	918	0	22.0	4.0	18	76%
<1.0	8.0	694	0	36.0	5.8	21	90%
<1.0	26.0	600	0	8.0	1.2	0	41%
<1.0	2.0	810	0	2.0	<1.0	0	72%
<1.0	12.0	700	(tr)	30.0	5.0	23	87%
<1.0	2.0	27	(mq)	<1.0	<1.0	0	0%
15.0	34.0	1003	(mq)	24.0	10.8	126	53%
10.0	22.0	669	(mq)	16.0	7.2	84	53%
0.0	48.0	19	0	0.0	0.0	0	0%
0.0	<1.0	35	0	0.0	0.0	0	0%
0.0	49.0	24	0	0.0	0.0	0	0%
0.0	61.0	27	0	0.0	0.0	0	0%
0.0	48.0	61	0	0.0	0.0	0	0%
14.0	42.0	891	(mq)	25.0	6.9	36	50%
29.0	49.0	1050	(mq)	23.0	5.0	66	40%
<1.0	11.0	160	0	<1.0	<1.0	<1	0%
0.0	30.0	6	0	0.0	0.0	0	0%
7.0	15.0	414	(mq)	11.0	3.7	18	53%
12.0	22.0	718	(mq)	17.0	5.9	29	54%
16.0	40.0	467	(mq)	16.0	5.6	37	40%
22.0	56.0	654	(mq)	22.0	7.9	52	39%

Food Name	Serving Size	Total Calories
TORTILLA CHIPS	1 oz	139
VEGETABLE OIL SPREAD, 'Country Crock'	.2 oz	25

KENTUCKY FRIED CHICKEN

Food Name	Serving Size	Total Calories
BARBECUE SAUCE	1 oz	35
BEANS		
barbecue baked	3.9 oz	132
green	3.6 oz	36
BISCUIT		
buttermilk, 2.3 oz	1 biscuit	232
regular, 2.0 oz	1 biscuit	200
BREADSTICKS, 1.2 oz	1 breadstick	110
CHICKEN		
breast, center, 'Extra Tasty Crispy' 4.8 oz	1 serving	342
breast, center, 'Hot & Spicy' 4.3 oz	1 serving	382
breast, center, 'Original Recipe' 3.6 oz	1 serving	260
breast, center, 'Skinfree Crispy'	1 serving	296
breast, side, 'Extra Tasty Crispy' 3.9 oz	1 serving	343
breast, side, 'Hot & Spicy' 4.1 oz	1 serving	398
breast, side, 'Original Recipe'	1 piece	276
breast, side, 'Skinfree Crispy'	1 serving	293
dark meat quarter, w/skin, 'Rotisserie Gold' 5.1 oz	1 serving	333
dark meat quarter, w/o skin, 'Rotisserie Gold' 4.1 oz	1 serving	217
drumstick, 'Extra Tasty Crispy' 2.4 oz	1 serving	190
drumstick, 'Hot & Spicy' 2.3 oz	1 serving	190
drumstick, 'Original Recipe' 1.8 oz	1 piece	130
drumstick, 'Skinfree Crispy'	1 serving	166
'Hot Wings' 6 pieces, 4.8 oz	1 serving	471
'Spicy Chicken Bites' small 4.3 oz	1 serving	248

Prot. MGS	Carbs. GMS	Sodium MGS	Fiber GMS	Fat GMS	Sat. Fat GMS	Chol. MGS	% Fat Cal.
2.0	18.0	134	(mq)	6.0	na	<1	39%
0.0	0.0	40	(mq)	2.8	<1.0	0	100%
0.3	7.1	450	na	0.6	0.1	<1	15%
5.0	24.0	535	4.0	2.0	1.0	3	14%
1.0	5.0	563	2.0	1.0	0.0	3	27%
4.2	27.1	539	(mq)	11.9	2.8	1	46%
3.0	20.0	564	1.0	12.0	3.0	2	52%
3.0	17.0	15	0	3.0	0.0	0	25%
33.0	11.7	790	(mq)	19.7	4.8	114	52%
24.3	16.0	905	na	25.0	6.0	84	59%
25.0	8.0	609	na	14.0	4.0	na	48%
24.0	11.0	435	na	16.0	3.1	59	49%
21.7	14.0	748	(mq)	22.3	5.5	81	59%
20.5	18.0	922	na	27.0	7.0	83	61%
20.0	10.0	654	na	17.0	na	na	55%
22.0	11.0	410	na	17.0	3.5	63	52%
30.0	1.0	980	na	23.7	6.6	163	64%
27.0	0.0	772	na	12.2	3.5	128	51%
13.0	8.0	260	<1	11.0	3.0	60	53%
13.0	10.0	300	<1	11.0	3.0	50	53%
13.0	4.0	210	0	7.0	2.0	70	46%
13.0	8.0	256	na	9.0	1.9	42	49%
27.0	18.0	1230	na	33.0	8.0	150	63%
28.7	4.7	344	na	12.4	3.8	143	45%

Food Name	Serving Size	Total Calories
thigh, 'Extra Tasty Crispy' 4.2 oz	1 serving	370
thigh, 'Hot & Spicy' 3.8 oz	1 serving	370
thigh, 'Original Recipe' 3.3 oz	1 piece	260
thigh, 'Skinfree Crispy'	1 serving	256
white meat quarter, w/o skin and wing, 'Rotisserie Gold' 4.1 oz	1 serving	199
white meat quarter, w/skin and wing, 'Rotisserie Gold' 6.2 oz	1 serving	335
wing, 'Extra Tasty Crispy' 1.9 oz	1 serving	200
wing, 'Hot & Spicy' 1.9 oz	1 serving	210
wing, 'Original Recipe' 1.7 oz	1 piece	150
CHICKEN NUGGETS		
'Kentucky Nuggets' .6 oz	1 nugget	46
'Kentucky Nuggets' 3.4 oz	6 nuggets	284
CHICKEN SANDWICH		
'Chicken Littles'	1.7 oz	169
'Colonel's'	5.9 oz	482
'Value BBQ Flavored'	5.3 oz	256
COLESLAW	3.2 oz	114
CORN, on the cob	5.3 oz	222
CORNBREAD, 2 oz	1 serving	228
FRENCH FRIES		
'Crispy' 2.5 oz	1 serving	210
'Kentucky Fries'	1 serving	268
regular, 2.7 oz	1 serving	244
GRAVY, chicken	1 serving	59
HONEY SAUCE	.5 oz	49
MACARONI AND CHEESE	4 oz	162
MUSTARD SAUCE	1 oz	36
POTATO WEDGES	3.3 oz	192
POTATOES, MASHED		
plain	1 serving	59
w/gravy	4.2 oz	109

Prot. MGS	Carbs. GMS	Sodium MGS	Fiber GMS	Fat GMS	Sat. Fat GMS	Chol. MGS	% Fat Cal.
19.0	7.0	540	2.0	25.0	6.0	70	59%
18.0	13.0	570	1.0	27.0	7.0	90	65%
19.0	9.0	570	1.0	17.0	5.0	110	58%
17.0	9.0	394	na	17.0	3.6	68	60%
37.0	0.0	667	na	5.9	1.7	97	27%
40.0	1.0	1104	na	18.7	5.4	157	50%
10.0	10.0	290	<1	13.0	4.0	45	60%
10.0	9.0	340	<1	15.0	4.0	50	62%
11.0	7.0	380	0	8.0	3.0	40	53%
2.8	2.2	140	(mq)	2.9	0.7	12	57%
16.0	15.0	865	na	18.0	4.0	66	57%
5.7	13.8	331	(mq)	10.1	2.0	18	54%
20.8	38.6	1060	(mq)	27.3	5.7	47	51%
17.0	28.0	782	2.0	8.0	1.0	57	29%
1.0	13.0	177	na	6.0	1.0	<5	47%
4.0	27.0	76	8.0	12.0	2.0	0	49%
3.0	25.0	194	1.0	13.0	2.0	42	51%
3.0	24.0	493	3.0	11.0	3.0	4	47%
5.0	33.0	81	na	13.0	na	na	44%
3.2	31.1	139	(mq)	11.9	2.6	2	44%
2.0	4.0	398	na	4.0	na	na	61%
0.0	12.1	15	0	<.1	<.1	<1	<2%
7.0	15.0	531	0	8.0	3.0	16	46%
0.9	6.0	346	na	0.9	0.1	<1	23%
3.0	25.0	428	3.0	9.0	3.0	3	42%
2.0	12.0	228	na	tr	na	na	0%
1.0	16.0	386	2.0	5.0	<1.0	<1	41%

Food Name	Serving Size	Total Calories
RED BEANS AND RICE	3.9 oz	114
RICE, garden	3.8 oz	75
ROLL, sourdough, 1.7 oz	1 roll	128
SALAD		
garden	3.1 oz	16
macaroni	3.8 oz	248
pasta	3.8 oz	135
potato	4.4 oz	180
vegetable medley	4 oz	126
SALAD DRESSING		
Italian	1 oz	15
ranch	1 oz	170
SWEET AND SOUR SAUCE	1 oz	58

KRYSTAL

BISCUIT	3.2 oz	289
BREAKFAST, gravy biscuit	8.2 oz	445
BREAKFAST SANDWICH		
bacon biscuit	3.6 oz	355
country ham biscuit	4.5 oz	379
egg biscuit	4.8 oz	372
sausage biscuit	4.3 oz	429
CHEESEBURGER		
bacon	6.4 oz	583
'Burger Plus'	7 oz	545
double	1 serving	214
regular	1 serving	189
CHICKEN SANDWICH	6.4 oz	392
CHILI		
large, 12 oz	1 serving	322
regular, 8 oz	1 serving	214

Prot. MGS	Carbs. GMS	Sodium MGS	Fiber GMS	Fat GMS	Sat. Fat GMS	Chol. MGS	% Fat Cal.
4.0	18.0	315	3.0	3.0	1.0	4	23%
2.0	15.0	576	1.0	1.0	0.0	0	11%
4.0	24.0	236	1.0	2.0	0.0	0	14%
1.0	3.0	10	1.0	0.0	0.0	0	0%
4.0	20.0	6	1.0	17.0	3.0	12	62%
2.0	14.0	663	1.0	8.0	1.0	1	53%
3.0	18.0	423	2.0	11.0	2.0	11	55%
1.0	21.0	240	3.0	4.0	1.0	0	29%
0.0	2.0	420	0	1.0	0.0	0	60%
0.0	1.0	250	0	18.0	3.0	10	95%
0.1	13.0	148	na	0.6	0.1	<1	9%
5.0	35.0	777	na	14.0	3.0	1	44%
9.0	43.0	1306	na	26.0	5.0	13	53%
9.0	36.0	1055	na	20.0	5.0	14	51%
15.0	36.0	1488	na	19.0	5.0	23	45%
10.0	36.0	813	na	21.0	5.0	133	51%
10.0	37.0	987	na	27.0	7.0	29	57%
36.0	34.0	935	na	35.0	14.0	114	54%
33.0	37.0	962	na	31.0	12.0	105	51%
11.0	22.0	674	na	8.0	2.0	16	34%
11.0	16.0	456	na	10.0	4.0	30	48%
21.0	44.0	707	na	16.0	na	33	37%
17.0	33.0	1012	na	11.0	na	25	31%
11.0	22.0	674	na	8.0	na	16	34%

Food Name	Serving Size	Total Calories
DONUT		
plain	1.3 oz	100
w/chocolate icing	1.8 oz	162
w/vanilla icing	1.8 oz	148
FRENCH FRIES		
'Krys Kross'	2.6 oz	242
'Krys Kross' w/cheese	3.6 oz	292
large order, 5 oz	1 serving	615
medium order, 3.9 oz	1 serving	474
small order, 2.8 oz	1 serving	338
HAMBURGER		
'Big K'	7.3 oz	608
'Burger Plus'	6.4 oz	488
double, 4 oz	1 serving	276
small, 2.2 oz	1 serving	158
HOT DOG		
'Chili Cheese Pup'	2.6 oz	203
'Chili Pup'	2.5 oz	184
'Corn Pup'	2.3 oz	214
plain	1.9 oz	164
MILKSHAKE, chocolate	12.8 oz	271
PIE		
apple	4.5 oz	320
lemon meringue	4 oz	340
pecan	4 oz	450

LITTLE CAESARS

Food Name	Serving Size	Total Calories
BREAD, 'Crazy Bread'	1 serving	98
HAM AND CHEESE SANDWICH	1 serving	520
PIZZA		
'Baby Pan!Pan!'	1 serving	525
cheese, round 'Pizza!Pizza!' large pie	1 serving	169

Prot. MGS	Carbs. GMS	Sodium MGS	Fiber GMS	Fat GMS	Sat. Fat GMS	Chol. MGS	% Fat Cal.
1.0	17.0	130	na	9.0	2.0	6	81%
1.0	27.0	149	na	11.0	3.0	6	61%
1.0	29.0	130	na	9.0	2.0	6	55%
3.0	33.0	589	na	11.0	5.0	10	41%
4.0	35.0	789	na	15.0	6.0	11	46%
5.0	111.0	191	na	17.0	8.0	15	25%
4.0	86.0	147	na	13.0	6.0	12	25%
3.0	61.0	105	na	9.0	na	8	24%
40.0	35.0	1281	na	36.0	14.0	125	53%
30.0	36.0	709	na	27.0	9.0	90	50%
18.0	24.0	532	na	14.0	5.0	43	46%
9.0	15.0	339	na	7.0	na	21	40%
8.0	15.0	623	na	13.0	5.0	24	58%
7.0	14.0	593	na	12.0	4.0	19	59%
6.0	17.0	566	na	14.0	6.0	24	59%
6.0	14.0	469	na	10.0	4.0	15	55%
8.0	41.0	175	na	10.0	5.0	32	33%
3.0	45.0	420	na	14.0	4.0	0	39%
7.0	60.0	130	na	9.0	3.0	45	24%
5.0	61.0	290	na	24.0	6.0	55	48%
4.0	18.0	119	na	1.0	na	2	9%
28.0	55.0	1045	.5	21.0	(mq)	45	36%
28.0	53.0	1180	na	22.0	na	60	38%
11.0	18.0	240	na	6.0	na	15	32%

Food Name	Serving Size	Total Calories
cheese, round 'Pizza!Pizza!' medium pie	1 serving	154
cheese, round 'Pizza!Pizza!' small pie	1 serving	138
cheese, single slice, 2.2 oz	1 serving	170
cheese, square 'Pizza!Pizza!' large pie	1 serving	188
cheese, square 'Pizza!Pizza!' medium pie	1 serving	185
cheese, square 'Pizza!Pizza!' small pie	1 serving	188
pepperoni combination, single slice	1 serving	190
PIZZA ENTRÉE		
cheese pizza, w/individual tossed salad	1 serving	600
vegetable pizza, w/individual tossed salad	1 serving	640
SALAD		
antipasto, w/low-calorie dressing, 12 oz	1 serving	170
Greek, small	1 serving	85
Greek, w/low-calorie dressing, 11 oz	1 serving	140
tossed, small	1 serving	37
tossed, w/low-calorie dressing, 11 oz	1 serving	80
SAUCE, 'Crazy Sauce'	1 serving	63
SUBMARINE SANDWICH, Italian	1 serving	590
TUNA MELT SANDWICH	1 serving	700
TURKEY SANDWICH	1 serving	450
VEGETARIAN SANDWICH	1 serving	620

LONG JOHN SILVER'S

Food Name	Serving Size	Total Calories
BEANS, green, 3.5 oz	1 serving	20
BREADSTICKS, 1.2 oz	1 serving	110
BROWNIE, walnut, 3.4 oz	1 brownie	440
CATFISH ENTRÉE, fillet, w/fries, 2 hushpuppies, and coleslaw	1 serving	860
CATFISH FILLET, 2.7 oz	1 serving	203

Prot. MGS	Carbs. GMS	Sodium MGS	Fiber GMS	Fat GMS	Sat. Fat GMS	Chol. MGS	% Fat Cal.
10.0	16.0	220	na	5.0	na	15	29%
9.0	14.0	200	na	5.0	na	15	33%
9.0	20.0	285	.2	6.0	(mq)	10	32%
10.0	22.0	380	na	6.0	na	20	29%
10.0	22.0	370	na	6.0	na	20	29%
10.0	22.0	380	na	6.0	na	20	29%
10.0	20.0	340	.8	7.0	(mq)	15	33%
30.0	73.0	1605	3.0	21.0	(mq)	35	32%
34.0	76.0	1715	3.6	22.0	(mq)	40	31%
10.0	12.0	1145	(mq)	9.0	(mq)	40	48%
4.0	6.0	400	na	5.0	na	10	53%
8.0	8.0	1075	(mq)	8.0	(mq)	25	51%
2.0	7.0	85	na	1.0	na	0	24%
4.0	11.0	745	(mq)	2.0	(mq)	0	23%
3.0	11.0	360	na	1.0	na	0	14%
29.0	55.0	1230	1.7	28.0	(mq)	60	43%
34.0	58.0	825	.6	37.0	(mq)	65	48%
24.0	49.0	1590	na	17.0	na	45	34%
30.0	58.0	1000	1.3	30.0	(mq)	55	44%
1.0	3.0	320	na	<1.0	<.3	0	0%
3.0	18.0	120	na	3.0	na	0	25%
5.0	54.0	150	na	22.0	5.4	20	45%
28.0	90.0	990	na	42.0	10.0	65	44%
12.0	13.0	469	na	12.0	na	na	53%

Food Name	Serving Size	Total Calories
CHEESECAKE, pineapple cream .... 3.2 oz		310
CHICKEN		
light herb, 3.5 oz .... 1 serving		120
'Plank' 1 piece .... 2 oz		120
'Planks' 2 pieces .... 4 oz		240
'Planks' 2 pieces, w/fries, hushpuppies,		
coleslaw .... 6.9 oz		490
CHICKEN ENTRÉE		
'Kids Meal' 2 pieces, w/fries, hushpuppy .. 7.8 oz		560
'Planks' 3 pieces, w/fries, hushpuppies,		
coleslaw .... 14.1 oz		890
'Planks' 4 pieces, w/fries, coleslaw ... 1 serving		940
w/rice, green beans, coleslaw, roll		
w/o margarine .... 15.9 oz		590
CHICKEN SANDWICH		
1 piece, batter-dipped, w/o sauce,		
4.5 oz .... 1 serving		280
CHOWDER		
clam, w/cod .... 1 serving		140
seafood, w/cod, 7 oz .... 1 serving		140
CLAM ENTRÉE, w/fries, hushpuppies,		
coleslaw .... 12.7 oz		990
CLAMS, breaded, 4.7 oz .... 1 serving		526
COLESLAW .... 1 serving		140
COMBINATION ENTRÉE		
fish, scallops, w/fries, 2 hushpuppies,		
coleslaw .... 1 serving		970
'Fish, Shrimp & Chicken' w/fries,		
hushpuppies, coleslaw .... 18.1 oz		1160
'Fish, Shrimp & Clams' w/fries,		
hushpuppies, coleslaw .... 18.1 oz		1240
'Fish & Chicken' w/fries, hushpuppies,		
coleslaw .... 15.2 oz		950

Prot. MGS	Carbs. GMS	Sodium MGS	Fiber GMS	Fat GMS	Sat. Fat GMS	Chol. MGS	% Fat Cal.
4.0	34.0	105	na	18.0	9.0	10	52%
22.0	<1.0	570	na	4.0	1.2	60	30%
8.0	11.0	400	na	3.0	1.6	15	23%
16.0	22.0	790	na	12.0	3.2	30	45%
19.0	50.0	1290	na	26.0	5.7	30	48%
21.0	60.0	1310	na	29.0	6.3	30	47%
32.0	101.0	2000	na	44.0	9.5	55	44%
39.0	94.0	1390	na	44.0	10.0	70	42%
32.0	82.0	1620	na	15.0	3.3	75	23%
14.0	39.0	790	na	8.0	2.1	15	26%
11.0	10.0	590	na	6.0	2.0	20	39%
11.0	10.0	590	na	6.0	1.8	20	39%
24.0	114.0	1830	na	52.0	10.9	75	47%
17.0	48.0	1170	na	31.0	na	na	53%
1.0	20.0	260	na	6.0	1.0	15	39%
30.0	109.0	1540	na	46.0	10.0	70	43%
45.0	113.0	2590	na	65.0	14.2	135	50%
44.0	123.0	2630	na	70.0	15.2	140	51%
36.0	102.0	2090	na	49.0	10.6	75	46%

Food Name	Serving Size	Total Calories
'Fish & Chicken Kids Meal' w/fries, hushpuppies	8.9 oz	620
'Fish & Shrimp' w/fries, hushpuppies, coleslaw	17.2 oz	1140
1 piece fish, 1 piece chicken, w/fries	8.1 oz	550
COOKIE		
chocolate chip	1.8 oz	230
oatmeal raisin	1.8 oz	160
CORN, cobbette, 3.3 oz	1 cob	140
CRACKER, saltine, 1 pkg	2 crackers	25
FISH. See also individual listings.		
baked, w/sauce, 5.5 oz	1 serving	151
batter-dipped, 1 piece	3.1 oz	180
crispy, 1.8 oz	1 serving	150
kitchen breaded, 2 oz	1 serving	122
lemon crumb, 3 pieces, 5 oz	1 serving	150
light paprika, 3 pieces, 4.7 oz	1 serving	120
scampi sauce, 3 pieces, 5.2 oz	1 serving	170
FISH ENTRÉE. See also individual listings.		
baked, w/sauce, coleslaw, mixed vegetables	1 serving	387
'Crispy Fish' 3 pieces, w/fries, hushpuppies, coleslaw	13.5 oz	980
'Fish & Fries Kids Meal' 1 piece, w/fries, hushpuppy, 7 oz	1 serving	500
'Fish & Fries' 3 pieces, w/ fries, 2 hushpuppies	1 serving	810
'Fish & Fries' 2 pieces, w/ fries, 9.2 oz	1 serving	610
'Fish & More' 2 pieces, w/fries, hushpuppies, coleslaw	14.4 oz	890
'Homestyle' 6 pieces, w/fries, 2 hushpuppies, coleslaw	1 serving	1260

Prot. MGS	Carbs. GMS	Sodium MGS	Fiber GMS	Fat GMS	Sat. Fat GMS	Chol. MGS	% Fat Cal.
24.0	61.0	1400	na	34.0	7.4	45	49%
40.0	108.0	2440	na	65.0	14.1	145	51%
23.0	51.0	1380	na	32.0	6.8	45	52%
3.0	35.0	170	na	9.0	5.7	10	35%
3.0	15.0	150	na	10.0	2.0	15	56%
3.0	18.0	0	na	8.0	na	0	51%
<1.0	4.0	75	na	1.0	na	0	36%
33.0	0.0	361	na	2.0	na	na	12%
12.0	12.0	490	na	11.0	2.7	30	55%
8.0	8.0	240	na	8.0	2.2	20	48%
9.0	8.0	374	na	5.0	na	na	37%
29.0	4.0	370	na	1.0	na	110	6%
28.0	<1.0	120	na	<1.0	na	110	<7%
28.0	2.0	270	na	5.0	na	110	26%
36.0	19.0	1298	na	19.0	na	na	44%
31.0	92.0	1530	na	50.0	11.3	70	46%
16.0	50.0	1010	na	28.0	5.8	30	50%
42.0	77.0	1630	na	38.0	9.0	85	42%
27.0	52.0	1480	na	37.0	7.9	60	55%
31.0	92.0	1790	na	48.0	10.1	75	49%
49.0	124.0	1590	na	64.0	14.0	130	46%

Food Name	Serving Size	Total Calories
kitchen breaded, 3 pieces, w/fries, hushpuppies, coleslaw	1 serving	940
kitchen breaded, 2 pieces, w/fries, hushpuppies, coleslaw	1 serving	818
lemon crumb, 2 pieces, w/rice, salad, 'Light' 11.8 oz	1 serving	290
light paprika, 2 pieces, w/rice and small salad	10 oz	300
3 pieces, w/fries, 2 hushpuppies, coleslaw	1 serving	960
3 pieces, w/rice, green bean, coleslaw, roll w/o butter	17.4 oz	610
FISH SANDWICH		
'Homestyle'	1 serving	510
'Homestyle Platter' w/fries, coleslaw ..	1 serving	870
1 piece, batter-dipped, w/o sauce, 5.6 oz	1 serving	340
FRENCH FRIES, 3 oz	1 serving	220
HONEY MUSTARD SAUCE	1 oz	56
HUSHPUPPY	1 piece	70
MALT VINEGAR	1 oz	1
MIXED VEGETABLES, 4 oz	1 serving	60
OYSTER ENTRÉE, 6 pieces, w/fries and coleslaw	1 serving	789
OYSTERS, 3 pieces, breaded, 2.1 oz ...	1 serving	180
PIE		
apple	4.5 oz	320
cherry	4.5 oz	360
lemon	4 oz	340
pecan	4 oz	446
pumpkin	4 oz	251
RICE PILAF, 5 oz	1 serving	210
ROLL	1.5 oz	110

Prot. MGS	Carbs. GMS	Sodium MGS	Fiber GMS	Fat GMS	Sat. Fat GMS	Chol. MGS	% Fat Cal.
35.0	84.0	1900	na	52.0	na	na	50%
26.0	76.0	1526	na	46.0	na	na	51%
24.0	40.0	690	na	5.0	na	75	16%
24.0	45.0	650	na	2.0	na	70	6%
43.0	97.0	1890	na	44.0	10.0	100	41%
39.0	86.0	1420	na	13.0	2.2	125	19%
22.0	58.0	780	na	22.0	5.0	48	39%
26.0	108.0	1110	na	38.0	8.0	55	39%
18.0	40.0	890	na	13.0	3.2	30	34%
3.0	30.0	60	na	10.0	3.0	5	41%
tr	14.0	315	na	tr	na	na	0%
2.0	10.0	25	na	2.0	1.0	5	26%
0.0	0.0	15	na	0.0	0.0	na	0%
2.0	9.0	330	na	2.0	1.0	0	30%
17.0	78.0	763	na	45.0	na	na	51%
6.0	18.0	195	na	9.0	na	na	45%
3.0	45.0	420	na	13.0	4.5	5	37%
4.0	55.0	200	na	13.0	4.4	5	33%
7.0	60.0	130	na	9.0	3.0	45	24%
5.0	59.0	435	na	22.0	na	na	44%
4.0	34.0	242	na	11.0	na	na	39%
5.0	43.0	570	na	2.0	na	0	9%
4.0	23.0	170	na	<1.0	<.3	0	<8%

Food Name	Serving Size	Total Calories
SALAD		
garden, w/crackers	1 serving	170
ocean chef, w/crackers	1 serving	250
ocean chef, w/o dressing or crackers, 8.3 oz	1 serving	110
seafood, 1 scoop	1 serving	210
seafood, w/crackers	1 serving	270
seafood, w/o dressing or crackers, 9.8 oz	1 serving	380
shrimp, w/crackers	1 serving	183
small, w/o dressing, 1.9 oz	1 serving	8
SALAD DRESSING		
blue cheese	1.5 oz	225
Italian, reduced calorie	1.5 oz	20
sea salad	1.5 oz	220
Thousand Island	1.5 oz	225
SCALLOP ENTRÉE, w/fries and coleslaw	1 serving	747
SCALLOPS, battered, 3 pieces, 2.1 oz	1 serving	159
SEAFOOD GUMBO, w/cod	7 oz	120
SEAFOOD SAUCE	1 oz	34
SHRIMP		
batter-dipped, .4 oz	1 piece	30
breaded, 4.7 oz	1 serving	388
SHRIMP ENTRÉE		
breaded, 21 pieces, w/fries, hushpuppies, coleslaw	1 serving	1070
10 pieces, w/fries, hushpuppies, coleslaw	11.7 oz	840
w/scampi sauce	5.2 oz	120
SWEET AND SOUR SAUCE	.42 oz	20
TARTAR SAUCE	1 oz	117

Prot. MGS	Carbs. GMS	Sodium MGS	Fiber GMS	Fat GMS	Sat. Fat GMS	Chol. MGS	% Fat Cal.
9.0	13.0	380	na	9.0	2.0	5	48%
24.0	19.0	1340	na	9.0	1.0	80	32%
12.0	13.0	730	na	1.0	0.4	40	8%
14.0	26.0	570	na	5.0	1.0	90	21%
16.0	36.0	670	na	7.0	1.0	90	23%
15.0	12.0	980	na	31.0	5.1	55	73%
27.0	12.0	658	na	3.0	na	na	15%
<1.0	2.0	0	na	0.0	na	0	0%
2.0	3.0	na	na	23.0	na	na	92%
tr	3.0	882	na	1.0	na	na	45%
2.0	5.0	na	na	21.0	na	na	86%
tr	8.0	422	na	22.0	na	na	88%
17.0	66.0	1579	na	45.0	na	na	54%
6.0	12.0	503	na	9.0	na	na	51%
9.0	4.0	740	na	8.0	2.1	25	60%
tr	9.0	357	na	tr	na	na	0%
1.0	2.0	80	na	2.0	0.5	10	60%
12.0	33.0	1229	na	23.0	na	na	53%
25.0	130.0	1790	na	51.0	11.0	125	43%
18.0	88.0	1630	na	47.0	9.7	100	50%
15.0	2.0	610	na	5.0	na	205	38%
<1.0	5.0	45	na	<1.0	<.3	0	0%
tr	5.0	228	na	11.0	na	na	85%

Food Name	Serving Size	Total Calories

MAZZIO'S PIZZA

Food Name	Serving Size	Total Calories
BEEF SANDWICH, barbecue beef and cheddar	1 sandwich	580
CHICKEN SANDWICH, chicken and cheddar	1 sandwich	570
GARLIC BREAD, w/cheese	2 slices	700
HAM AND CHEESE SANDWICH	1 sandwich	790
LASAGNA, meat, small	1 serving	460
NACHOS, w/meat	4.5 oz	500
PASTA AND NOODLES		
chicken parmesan	17.5 oz	590
fettuccine Alfredo, small	1 serving	440
spaghetti, small	1 serving	290
PIZZA		
cheese, deep pan	1 slice	350
cheese, original crust, medium pie	1 slice	260
cheese, thin crust	1 slice	220
combo, deep pan, medium pie	1 slice	410
combo, original crust, medium pie	1 slice	320
'Light' medium pie	1 slice	240
pepperoni, deep pan, medium pie	1 slice	380
pepperoni, original crust, medium pie	1 slice	280
sausage, deep pan, medium pie	1 slice	430
sausage, original crust, medium pie	1 slice	350
SUBMARINE SANDWICH, 'Deluxe'	1 sandwich	810

MC DONALD'S

Food Name	Serving Size	Total Calories
APPLE JUICE	6 oz	80
APPLE PIE, 3.0 oz	1 serving	260
BACON BITS	1 oz	15
BARBECUE SAUCE	1 serving	50

Prot. MGS	Carbs. GMS	Sodium MGS	Fiber GMS	Fat GMS	Sat. Fat GMS	Chol. MGS	% Fat Cal.
39.0	53.0	1260	na	24.0	11.0	95	37%
33.0	56.0	1350	na	24.0	8.0	70	38%
21.0	74.0	1280	na	35.0	7.0	15	45%
40.0	71.0	1900	na	39.0	13.0	85	44%
24.0	26.0	1370	na	25.0	10.0	95	49%
21.0	21.0	1200	na	37.0	17.0	75	67%
39.0	68.0	1600	na	19.0	3.0	50	29%
14.0	34.0	680	na	28.0	16.0	55	57%
11.0	39.0	800	na	10.0	na	5	31%
17.0	42.0	620	na	8.0	na	15	21%
14.0	33.0	450	na	8.0	na	10	28%
13.0	22.0	440	na	9.0	na	15	37%
19.0	42.0	930	na	18.0	6.0	20	40%
17.0	34.0	780	na	13.0	6.0	25	37%
10.0	30.0	460	na	8.0	4.0	20	30%
18.0	38.0	740	na	17.0	6.0	25	40%
16.0	30.0	600	na	11.0	5.0	30	35%
21.0	41.0	1040	na	21.0	8.0	25	44%
18.0	34.0	890	na	16.0	7.0	20	41%
39.0	68.0	2240	na	43.0	13.0	75	48%
0.0	21.0	30	na	0.0	0.0	0	0%
2.0	30.0	240	(mq)	15.0	10.0	6	52%
1.0	0.0	95	na	1.0	0.3	1	60%
0.0	12.0	340	0	0.5	0.2	0	9%

Food Name	Serving Size	Total Calories
BISCUIT, w/spread, 2.6 oz	1 serving	260
BREAKFAST		
Cheerios cereal, w/o milk, 3/4 cup	1 serving	80
eggs, scrambled, 3.5 oz	1 serving	140
hotcakes, w/margarine and syrup, 6.2 oz	1 serving	440
sausage, 1.5 oz	1 serving	160
Wheaties cereal, w/o milk, 3/4 cup . . .	1 serving	90
BREAKFAST SANDWICH		
biscuit, bacon, egg, and cheese, 5.4 oz	1 serving	440
biscuit, sausage and egg, 6.2 oz	1 serving	505
biscuit, sausage, 4.2 oz	1 serving	420
egg, ham, and cheese, 'Egg McMuffin' 4.8 oz	1 serving	280
sausage, 'Sausage McMuffin' 4.8 oz . .	1 serving	345
sausage, 'Sausage Egg McMuffin' 5.6 oz	1 serving	430
CHEESEBURGER		
'McLean Deluxe' 7.7 oz	1 serving	370
'Quarter Pounder' 6.8 oz	1 serving	510
regular, 4.1 oz	1 serving	305
CHICKEN NUGGET, 'Chicken McNuggets' 6 pieces	1 serving	270
CHICKEN SANDWICH, 'McChicken' 6.6 oz	1 serving	415
CHOW MEIN NOODLES	1 serving	45
COOKIE		
'Chocolaty Chip' 2 oz	1 serving	330
'McDonaldland' 2 oz	1 serving	290
CROUTONS	.4 oz	50
DANISH		
apple, 4.1 oz	1 serving	390
cinnamon raisin, 3.9 oz	1 serving	440

Prot. MGS	Carbs. GMS	Sodium MGS	Fiber GMS	Fat GMS	Sat. Fat GMS	Chol. MGS	% Fat Cal.
5.0	32.0	730	(mq)	13.0	9.0	1	45%
3.0	14.0	210	na	1.0	0.4	0	11%
12.0	1.0	290	0	10.0	5.0	425	64%
8.0	74.0	685	(mq)	12.0	5.0	8	25%
7.0	0.0	310	0	15.0	5.0	43	84%
2.0	19.0	220	na	1.0	0.2	0	10%
15.0	33.0	1215	(mq)	26.0	16.0	240	53%
19.0	33.0	1210	(mq)	33.0	20.0	260	59%
12.0	32.0	1040	(mq)	28.0	17.0	44	60%
18.0	28.0	710	(mq)	11.0	4.0	235	35%
15.0	27.0	770	(mq)	20.0	11.0	57	52%
21.0	27.0	920	(mq)	25.0	14.0	270	52%
24.0	35.0	890	(mq)	14.0	8.0	75	34%
28.0	34.0	1110	(mq)	28.0	16.0	115	49%
15.0	30.0	725	(mq)	13.0	7.0	50	38%
20.0	17.0	580	(mq)	15.0	10.0	55	50%
19.0	39.0	830	(mq)	19.0	9.0	50	41%
1.0	5.0	60	na	2.0	1.0	2	40%
4.0	42.0	280	(mq)	15.0	10.0	4	41%
4.0	47.0	300	(mq)	9.0	7.0	0	28%
1.0	7.0	140	(mq)	2.0	1.3	0	36%
6.0	51.0	370	(mq)	17.0	11.0	25	39%
6.0	58.0	430	(mq)	21.0	13.0	34	43%

Food Name	Serving Size	Total Calories
cheese, iced, 3.9 oz . . . . 1 serving		390
raspberry, 4.1 oz . . . . 1 serving		410
ENGLISH MUFFIN, w/spread, 2.1 oz . . . . 1 muffin		170
FISH SANDWICH, 'Fillet-O-Fish' 5 oz . . . 1 serving		370
FRENCH FRIES		
large order . . . . 4.3 oz		400
large order, unsalted . . . . 4.3 oz		400
medium order . . . . 3.4 oz		320
medium order, unsalted . . . . 3.4 oz		320
small order . . . . 2.4 oz		220
small order, unsalted . . . . 2.4 oz		220
GRAPEFRUIT JUICE . . . . 6 oz		80
HAMBURGER		
'Big Mac' 7.6 oz . . . . 1 serving		500
'McLean Deluxe' 7.3 oz . . . . 1 serving		320
'Quarter Pounder' 5.9 oz . . . . 1 serving		410
regular, 3.6 oz . . . . 1 serving		255
HAMBURGER PATTY, 'McLean Deluxe'		
3 oz . . . . 1 serving		130
HONEY SAUCE . . . . 1 serving		45
MILK, 1% . . . . 8 oz		110
MILKSHAKE		
chocolate, low-fat . . . . 10.4 oz		320
strawberry, low-fat . . . . 10.4 oz		320
vanilla, low-fat . . . . 10.4 oz		290
MUFFIN		
apple bran, fat-free, 2.6 oz . . . . 1 muffin		180
blueberry, fat-free, 2.6 oz . . . . 1 muffin		170
MUSTARD SAUCE, hot . . . . 1 serving		70
ORANGE JUICE . . . . 6 oz		80
POTATOES, HASH BROWN 1.9 oz . . . . 1 serving		130
SALAD		
chef's, 9.5 oz . . . . 1 serving		170

Prot. MGS	Carbs. GMS	Sodium MGS	Fiber GMS	Fat GMS	Sat. Fat GMS	Chol. MGS	% Fat Cal.
7.0	42.0	420	(mq)	21.0	13.0	47	48%
6.0	62.0	310	(mq)	16.0	11.0	26	35%
5.0	26.0	285	(mq)	4.0	2.0	0	21%
14.0	38.0	730	(mq)	18.0	8.0	50	44%
6.0	46.0	200	(mq)	22.0	15.0	0	50%
6.0	46.0	45	(mq)	22.0	15.0	0	50%
4.0	36.0	150	(mq)	17.0	12.0	0	48%
4.0	36.0	35	(mq)	17.0	12.0	0	48%
3.0	26.0	110	(mq)	12.0	8.0	0	49%
3.0	26.0	25	(mq)	12.0	8.0	0	49%
1.0	19.0	0	na	0.0	0.0	0	0%
25.0	42.0	890	(mq)	26.0	16.0	100	47%
22.0	35.0	670	(mq)	10.0	5.0	60	28%
23.0	34.0	645	(mq)	20.0	11.0	85	44%
12.0	30.0	490	(mq)	9.0	5.0	37	32%
17.0	0.0	110	0	7.0	3.0	60	48%
0.0	12.0	0	0	0.0	0.0	0	0%
9.0	12.0	130	na	2.0	0.3	10	16%
11.0	66.0	240	(tr)	1.7	0.9	10	5%
11.0	67.0	170	(tr)	1.3	0.6	10	4%
11.0	60.0	170	0	1.3	0.6	10	4%
5.0	40.0	200	(mq)	0.0	0.0	0	0%
3.0	40.0	220	na	0.0	0.0	0	0%
0.0	8.0	250	0	3.6	1.2	5	46%
1.0	19.0	0	na	0.0	0.0	0	0%
1.0	15.0	330	(mq)	7.0	4.0	0	48%
17.0	8.0	400	(mq)	9.0	4.0	111	48%

Food Name	Serving Size	Total Calories
chunky chicken, 9.0 oz	1 serving	150
garden, 6.7 oz	1 serving	50
side order, 3.7 oz	1 serving	30
SALAD DRESSING		
blue cheese, 1 tbsp	.5 oz	50
French, red, reduced calorie, 1 tbsp	.5 oz	40
Oriental	.5 oz	24
ranch, 1 tbsp	.5 oz	55
Thousand Island, 1 tbsp	.5 oz	78
vinaigrette, 1 tbsp	.5 oz	12
SOFT DRINK		
Coca-Cola Classic, extra large	32 oz	380
Coca-Cola Classic, large	22 oz	260
Coca-Cola Classic, medium	16 oz	190
Coca-Cola Classic, small	12 oz	140
Diet Coke, extra large	32 oz	3
Diet Coke, large	22 oz	2
Diet Coke, medium	16 oz	1
Diet Coke, small	12 oz	1
orange, extra large	32 oz	360
orange, large	22 oz	240
orange, medium	16 oz	180
orange, small	12 oz	130
Sprite, extra large	32 oz	380
Sprite, large	22 oz	260
Sprite, medium	16 oz	190
Sprite, small	12 oz	140
SWEET AND SOUR SAUCE	1 serving	60
YOGURT, FROZEN		
cone, vanilla, low-fat	3 oz	105
hot caramel sundae, low-fat	6 oz	270
hot fudge sundae, low-fat	6 oz	240
strawberry sundae, low-fat	6 oz	210

Prot. MGS	Carbs. GMS	Sodium MGS	Fiber GMS	Fat GMS	Sat. Fat GMS	Chol. MGS	% Fat Cal.
25.0	7.0	230	(mq)	4.0	2.0	78	24%
4.0	6.0	70	(mq)	2.0	1.0	65	36%
2.0	4.0	35	(mq)	1.0	0.5	33	30%
0.0	1.0	150	na	4.0	1.0	7	72%
0.0	5.0	115	na	2.0	0.5	0	45%
tr	6.0	180	na	tr	0.0	0	0%
0.0	1.0	130	na	5.0	0.5	5	82%
0.0	2.0	100	na	8.0	2.0	8	92%
0.0	2.0	60	na	0.5	0.1	0	38%
0.0	101.0	40	na	0.0	0.0	0	0%
0.0	70.0	25	na	0.0	0.0	0	0%
0.0	50.0	20	na	0.0	0.0	0	0%
0.0	38.0	15	na	0.0	0.0	0	0%
0.0	0.6	80	na	0.0	0.0	0	0%
0.0	0.5	60	na	0.0	0.0	0	0%
0.0	0.4	40	na	0.0	0.0	0	0%
0.0	0.3	30	na	0.0	0.0	0	0%
0.0	88.0	25	na	0.0	0.0	0	0%
0.0	60.0	20	na	0.0	0.0	0	0%
0.0	44.0	20	na	0.0	0.0	0	0%
0.0	33.0	10	na	0.0	0.0	0	0%
0.0	96.0	40	na	0.0	0.0	0	0%
0.0	66.0	25	na	0.0	0.0	0	0%
0.0	48.0	20	na	0.0	0.0	0	0%
0.0	36.0	15	na	0.0	0.0	0	0%
0.0	14.0	190	0	0.2	0.1	0	3%
4.0	22.0	80	(mq)	1.0	0.3	3	9%
7.0	59.0	180	(tr)	3.0	1.0	13	10%
7.0	50.0	170	(tr)	3.0	0.5	6	11%
6.0	49.0	170	(tr)	1.0	0.5	6	4%

Food Name	Serving Size	Total Calories

MRS. WINNER'S

BAKED BEANS	1 serving	149
BISCUIT	1 serving	245
BREAKFAST		
country ham	1 serving	60
sausage patty	1 serving	200
CHICKEN		
breast, fried, skin-free	4 oz	280
dark meat quarter, 'Rotisserie'	4 oz	216
fillet, baked	1 serving	120
leg, fried, skin-free	1.7 oz	110
white meat quarter, 'Rotisserie'	5 oz	242
CHICKEN SANDWICH		
breaded	1 serving	203
fillet	1 serving	379
salad	1 serving	313
COLESLAW	1 serving	188
FRENCH FRIES	1 serving	225
POTATO WEDGES, oven roasted	1 serving	139
POTATOES, MASHED, w/gravy	1 serving	148
ROLL, honey yeast	1 roll	200
SALAD		
chicken	1 serving	583
seafood	1 serving	553
tossed	1 serving	6
STEAK ENTRÉE, country-fried	1 serving	220
STEAK SANDWICH	1 serving	429

ORANGE JULIUS

JUICE DRINK		
orange, regular	16 oz	265

Prot. MGS	Carbs. GMS	Sodium MGS	Fiber GMS	Fat GMS	Sat. Fat GMS	Chol. MGS	% Fat Cal.
5.0	31.0	436	na	na	na	1	0%
4.0	45.0	503	na	5.0	na	tr	18%
4.0	tr	565	na	1.0	na	14	15%
6.0	tr	400	na	10.0	na	8	45%
23.0	14.0	480	na	15.0	na	115	48%
29.0	2.0	590	na	10.0	na	140	42%
10.0	tr	360	na	2.0	na	33	15%
10.0	5.0	115	na	6.0	na	50	49%
38.0	2.0	700	na	9.0	na	139	33%
19.0	12.0	1000	na	10.0	na	37	44%
12.0	45.0	541	na	7.0	na	28	17%
10.0	33.0	599	na	6.0	na	1	17%
1.0	9.0	549	na	16.0	na	1	77%
6.0	27.0	214	na	9.0	na	1	36%
4.0	31.0	132	na	1.0	na	1	6%
3.0	22.0	823	na	3.0	na	2	18%
8.0	35.0	290	na	4.0	na	7	18%
9.0	39.0	875	na	8.0	na	3	12%
5.0	41.0	756	na	9.0	na	4	15%
1.0	1.0	439	na	tr	na	1	0%
12.0	tr	205	na	14.0	na	7	57%
11.0	43.0	644	na	11.0	na	21	23%
1.0	66.0	15	na	1.0	na	na	3%

Food Name	Serving Size	Total Calories
pina colada, regular	16 oz	300
raspberry cream supreme, regular	16 oz	510
strawberry, regular	16 oz	340
tropical cream supreme, regular	16 oz	510

PERKINS

BROCCOLI, raw	4 oz	31
CARROTS, raw	4 oz	49
CAULIFLOWER, raw	4 oz	27
CHICKEN DINNER, lemon pepper, w/rice pilaf, broccoli, salad	1 serving	620
FISH DINNER, orange roughy, w/rice pilaf, broccoli, salad	1 serving	467
FRUIT CUP, cantaloupe, honeydew, blueberries, 4.5 oz	1 serving	48
MARGARINE	1 scant tbsp	60
MUFFIN		
apple, 6.5 oz pre-baked wt	1 muffin	543
banana nut, 6.5 oz pre-baked wt	1 muffin	586
blueberry, 6.5 oz pre-baked wt	1 muffin	506
bran, 6.5 oz pre-baked wt	1 muffin	478
carrot, 6.5 oz pre-baked wt	1 muffin	560
chocolate chocolate chip, 6.5 oz pre-baked wt	1 muffin	546
corn, 6.5 oz pre-baked wt	1 muffin	683
cranberry nut, 6.5 oz pre-baked wt	1 muffin	558
oat bran, 6.5 oz pre-baked wt	1 muffin	513
plain, 6.5 oz pre-baked wt	1 muffin	586
plain, 98% fat-free, 6.5 oz pre-baked wt	1 muffin	495
MUSHROOMS, raw	4 oz	29
OMELETTE		
country club	1 serving	932

Prot. MGS	Carbs. GMS	Sodium MGS	Fiber GMS	Fat GMS	Sat. Fat GMS	Chol. MGS	% Fat Cal.
2.0	71.0	15	na	1.0	na	na	3%
4.0	76.0	40	na	23.0	na	na	41%
1.0	82.0	15	na	1.0	na	na	3%
5.0	67.0	40	na	25.0	na	95	44%
3.4	5.9	31	na	0.4	na	0	12%
1.2	11.5	39	na	0.2	na	0	4%
2.2	5.6	16	na	0.2	na	0	7%
59.4	59.6	1364	na	12.5	na	136	18%
33.0	60.0	1387	na	7.0	na	133	13%
0.8	11.9	12	na	0.3	na	0	6%
0.0	0.0	60	na	6.5	na	0	98%
9.0	76.0	728	na	24.0	na	95	40%
9.0	75.0	702	na	29.0	na	92	45%
7.0	71.0	671	na	23.0	na	88	41%
9.0	83.0	572	na	17.0	na	0	32%
7.0	88.0	780	na	23.0	na	81	37%
10.0	73.0	629	na	26.0	na	83	43%
12.0	121.0	1550	na	17.0	na	33	22%
9.0	71.0	671	na	28.0	na	88	45%
10.0	87.0	588	na	16.0	na	0	28%
9.0	81.0	797	na	26.0	na	104	40%
11.8	111.0	802	na	1.2	na	5	2%
2.4	5.3	3	na	0.5	na	0	16%
47.2	5.8	1134	<1.0	79.1	na	1154	76%

Food Name	Serving Size	Total Calories
country club, w/3 oz hash browns	1 serving	1033
deli ham and cheese	1 serving	962
deli ham and cheese, w/3 oz hash browns	1 serving	1063
'Denver' w/fruit cup	1 serving	235
'Everything'	1 serving	697
'Everything' w/3 oz hash browns	1 serving	798
Granny's country	1 serving	941
Granny's country, w/9 oz hash browns	1 serving	1245
ham and cheese	1 serving	644
ham and cheese, w/3 oz hash browns	1 serving	745
mushroom and cheese	1 serving	687
mushroom and cheese, w/3 oz hash browns	1 serving	788
seafood, w/fruit cup	1 serving	271
ONION, raw	4 oz	38
PANCAKES		
buttermilk	3 pancakes	442
'Harvest Grain' w/1.5 oz low-calorie syrup	5 pancakes	473
'Short Stack Harvest Grain'	3 pancakes	268
PIE		
apple	1 slice	521
apple, w/Equal	1 slice	420
cherry	1 slice	571
cherry, w/Equal	1 slice	425
coconut cream	1 slice	437
French silk	1 slice	551
lemon meringue, ...	1 slice	395
peanut butter brownie	1 slice	455
pecan	1 slice	669
POTATOES, HASH BROWN	3 oz	101

Prot. MGS	Carbs. GMS	Sodium MGS	Fiber GMS	Fat GMS	Sat. Fat GMS	Chol. MGS	% Fat Cal.
48.7	22.5	1162	<1.0	81.7	na	1154	71%
53.4	8.2	1832	<1.0	79.1	na	864	74%
54.9	24.9	1860	<1.0	81.7	na	864	69%
23.0	22.3	795	na	6.5	na	154	25%
44.5	8.6	870	na	53.4	na	814	69%
46.0	25.3	898	<2.0	56.0	na	814	63%
42.9	6.9	786	<1.0	81.5	na	810	78%
47.5	56.9	869	<1.0	89.2	na	810	64%
40.9	2.6	832	0	51.3	na	743	72%
42.4	19.3	860	0	53.9	na	743	65%
32.0	4.9	925	<1.0	59.9	na	744	78%
33.5	21.6	953	<1.0	62.5	na	744	71%
28.6	27.5	595	na	5.7	na	197	19%
1.3	8.3	3	na	0.3	na	0	7%
13.1	69.6	988	na	12.0	na	24	24%
11.3	93.0	1640	na	3.4	na	0	6%
6.8	55.7	1020	na	2.0	na	0	7%
3.0	72.0	457	na	26.0	na	0	45%
3.0	55.0	371	na	24.0	na	0	51%
4.0	84.0	702	na	26.0	na	0	41%
4.0	55.0	513	na	24.0	na	0	51%
6.0	56.0	488	na	33.0	na	5	68%
4.0	59.0	478	na	37.0	na	53	60%
2.0	63.0	528	na	16.0	na	0	36%
9.0	44.0	436	na	35.0	na	29	69%
7.0	106.0	670	na	26.0	na	17	35%
1.5	16.7	28	na	2.6	na	na	23%

Food Name	Serving Size	Total Calories
SALAD		
chef's, mini	1 serving	214
dinner, 'Lite & Healthy'	1 serving	103
SYRUP, low-calorie	1.5 oz	26
TOAST, w/.5 oz margarine, .75 oz grape jelly	1 slice	219
VEGETABLE SANDWICH		
pita, stir-fry	1 serving	308
pita, stir-fry, w/coleslaw	1 serving	441
pita, stir-fry, w/coleslaw and pasta salad	1 serving	626
pita, stir-fry, w/pasta salad	1 serving	493
mixed vegetables	6 oz	49
ZUCCHINI, raw	4 oz	22

PETER PIPER PIZZA

Food Name	Serving Size	Total Calories
PIZZA		
Beef		
express lunch pizza	1 slice	165
extra large pie	1 slice	280
large pie	1 slice	296
medium pie	1 slice	222
small pie	1 slice	194
Cheese		
express lunch pizza	1 pie	608
express lunch pizza	1 slice	152
extra large pie	1 pie	3078
extra large pie	1 slice	257
large pie	1 pie	2159
large pie	1 slice	270
medium pie	1 pie	1622
medium pie	1 slice	203

Prot. MGS	Carbs. GMS	Sodium MGS	Fiber GMS	Fat GMS	Sat. Fat GMS	Chol. MGS	% Fat Cal.
22.9	6.8	643	na	11.0	na	55	46%
3.4	14.7	496	na	2.1	na	0	18%
0.0	6.6	0	na	0.0	na	na	0%
2.3	27.7	224	1.0	12.2	na	8	50%
43.7	41.1	752	na	9.2	na	26	27%
44.7	53.9	877	na	17.8	na	36	36%
49.0	62.9	1395	na	32.5	na	37	47%
48.0	50.1	1270	na	23.9	na	27	44%
2.9	10.3	23	na	0.4	na	0	7%
1.2	4.7	1	na	0.1	na	0	4%
9.0	21.0	257	na	5.0	na	13	27%
15.0	36.0	446	na	8.0	na	20	26%
15.0	39.0	482	na	8.0	na	20	24%
12.0	29.0	359	na	6.0	na	15	24%
10.0	25.0	319	na	5.0	na	14	23%
32.0	83.0	609	na	16.0	na	47	24%
8.0	21.0	152	na	4.0	na	12	24%
160.0	437.0	3113	na	73.0	na	211	21%
13.0	36.0	260	na	6.1	na	18	21%
111.5	311.4	2176	na	49.4	na	140	21%
14.0	39.0	271	na	6.2	na	18	21%
84.0	235.0	1614	na	37.0	na	105	21%
11.0	29.0	201	na	5.0	na	13	22%

Food Name	Serving Size	Total Calories
small pie .... 1 pie	1059
small pie .... 1 slice	177
w/black olives, large pie .... 1 serving	259
w/black olives, medium pie .... 1 serving	193
w/black olives, small pie .... 1 serving	171
w/green pepper, large pie .... 1 serving	245
w/green pepper, medium pie .... 1 serving	183
w/green pepper, small pie .... 1 serving	163
w/ham, large pie .... 1 serving	258
w/ham, medium pie .... 1 serving	194
w/ham, small pie .... 1 serving	172
w/jalapeño, large pie .... 1 serving	244
w/jalapeño, medium pie .... 1 serving	183
w/jalapeño, small pie .... 1 serving	163
w/mushroom, large pie .... 1 serving	245
w/mushroom, medium pie .... 1 serving	183
w/mushroom, small pie .... 1 serving	162
w/onion, large pie .... 1 serving	243
w/onion, medium pie .... 1 serving	183
w/onion, small pie .... 1 serving	162
w/pineapple, large pie .... 1 serving	246
w/pineapple, medium pie .... 1 serving	185
w/pineapple, small pie .... 1 serving	164
Salami		
express lunch pizza .... 1 slice	164
extra large pie .... 1 slice	273
large pie .... 1 slice	288
medium pie .... 1 slice	216
small pie .... 1 slice	189

Prot. MGS	Carbs. GMS	Sodium MGS	Fiber GMS	Fat GMS	Sat. Fat GMS	Chol. MGS	% Fat Cal.
60.0	152.0	1073	na	25.0	na	70	21%
9.0	25.0	179	na	4.0	na	12	20%
24.0	22.0	407	na	8.0	na	12	28%
18.0	17.0	303	na	6.0	na	9	28%
16.0	15.0	276	na	6.0	na	8	32%
24.0	22.0	339	na	7.0	na	12	26%
18.0	17.0	256	na	5.0	na	9	25%
16.0	15.0	283	na	4.0	na	8	22%
26.0	22.0	473	na	7.0	na	17	24%
19.0	16.0	356	na	6.0	na	13	28%
17.0	15.0	317	na	5.0	na	11	26%
24.0	22.0	424	na	7.0	na	12	26%
18.0	17.0	319	na	5.0	na	9	25%
16.0	15.0	283	na	4.0	na	8	22%
24.0	22.0	379	na	7.0	na	12	26%
18.0	17.0	283	na	5.0	na	9	25%
16.0	15.0	245	na	4.0	na	8	22%
24.0	22.0	341	na	7.0	na	12	26%
18.0	17.0	257	na	5.0	na	9	25%
16.0	15.0	228	na	4.0	na	8	22%
23.0	23.0	341	na	7.0	na	12	26%
18.0	17.0	256	na	5.0	na	8	24%
16.0	15.0	228	na	4.0	na	8	22%
9.0	21.0	199	na	5.0	na	15	27%
14.0	37.0	322	na	7.5	na	22	25%
15.0	39.0	342	na	8.0	na	23	25%
11.0	29.0	254	na	6.0	na	17	25%
8.0	25.0	223	na	5.0	na	15	24%

Food Name	Serving Size	Total Calories

PIZZA HUT

PIZZA
Beef
hand-tossed .... 1 slice   261
'Pan Pizza' medium pie .... 1 slice   288
'Thick 'n Chewy' 10-inch pie .... 3 slices   620
'Thin 'n Crispy' 10-inch pie .... 3 slices   490
Cheese
'Bigfoot' .... 1 slice   179
hand-tossed, medium pie .... 1 slice   253
'Pan Pizza' medium pie .... 1 slice   279
'Thick 'n Chewy' 10-inch pie .... 3 slices   560
'Thin 'n Crispy' medium pie .... 1 slice   223
'Thin 'n Crispy' 10-inch pie .... 3 slices   450
'Chunky Combo'
hand-tossed, medium pie .... 1 slice   280
'Pan Pizza' medium pie .... 1 slice   306
'Thin 'n Crispy' medium pie .... 1 slice   250
'Chunky Meat'
hand-tossed, medium pie .... 1 slice   325
'Pan Pizza' medium pie .... 1 slice   352
'Thin 'n Crispy' medium pie .... 1 slice   295
Italian sausage
hand-tossed, medium pie .... 1 slice   313
'Pan Pizza' medium pie .... 1 slice   399
'Thin 'n Crispy' medium pie .... 1 slice   282
'Meat Lovers'
hand-tossed, medium pie .... 1 slice   321
'Pan Pizza' medium pie .... 1 slice   347
'Thin 'n Crispy' medium pie .... 1 slice   297
Pepperoni
'Bigfoot' .... 1 slice   195

Prot. MGS	Carbs. GMS	Sodium MGS	Fiber GMS	Fat GMS	Sat. Fat GMS	Chol. MGS	% Fat Cal.
15.0	28.0	795	2.0	10.0	3.0	25	34%
10.0	27.0	675	3.0	18.0	3.0	25	56%
38.0	73.0	na	na	20.0	na	na	29%
29.0	51.0	na	na	19.0	na	na	35%
9.0	24.0	959	2.0	5.0	3.0	14	25%
15.0	27.0	593	2.0	9.0	4.0	25	32%
14.0	26.0	473	2.0	13.0	5.0	25	42%
34.0	71.0	na	na	14.0	na	na	23%
13.0	19.0	503	2.0	10.0	5.0	25	40%
25.0	54.0	na	na	15.0	na	na	30%
14.8	28.0	823	2.5	11.6	4.8	29	37%
13.8	26.0	703	2.5	15.5	5.2	29	46%
12.7	20.0	736	2.0	12.7	5.0	29	46%
16.8	28.0	970	2.6	16.0	6.0	40	44%
15.7	27.0	850	2.6	20.0	7.0	40	51%
14.7	20.0	882	2.2	17.0	6.0	40	52%
16.0	27.0	871	2.0	15.0	6.0	38	43%
15.0	26.0	751	2.0	24.0	6.0	38	54%
14.0	20.0	781	2.0	17.0	6.0	38	54%
16.0	28.0	1106	3.0	15.0	4.0	42	42%
15.0	27.0	986	3.0	23.0	5.0	42	60%
14.0	20.0	1068	2.0	16.0	4.0	44	48%
10.0	24.0	1022	2.0	7.0	3.0	17	32%

Food Name	Serving Size	Total Calories
hand-tossed, medium pie	1 slice	253
'Pan Pizza' medium pie	1 slice	280
'Personal Pan Pizza' 9-oz pie	1 pie	675
'Thick 'n Chewy' 10-inch pie	3 slices	560
'Thin 'n Crispy' medium pie	1 slice	230
'Thin 'n Crispy' 10-inch pie	3 slices	430
Pepperoni, mushroom, Italian sausage, 'Bigfoot'	1 slice	213
'Pepperoni Lovers'		
hand-tossed, medium pie	1 slice	335
'Pan Pizza' medium pie	1 slice	362
'Thin 'n Crispy' medium pie	1 slice	320
Pork		
hand-tossed	1 slice	270
'Pan Pizza'	1 slice	296
'Thick 'n Chewy' 10-inch pie	3 slices	640
'Thin 'n Crispy' medium pie	1 slice	240
'Thin 'n Crispy' 10-inch pie	3 slices	520
'Super Supreme'		
hand-tossed, medium pie	2 slices	463
hand-tossed, medium pie	1 slice	276
'Pan Pizza' medium pie	1 slice	302
'Thin 'n Crispy' medium pie	1 slice	253
'Supreme'		
hand-tossed, medium pie	1 slice	289
'Pan Pizza' medium pie	1 slice	315
'Personal Pan Pizza' 9.3-oz pie	1 pie	647
'Thick 'n Chewy' 10-inch pie	3 slices	640
'Thin 'n Crispy' medium pie	1 slice	262
'Thin 'n Crispy' 10-inch pie	3 slices	510
'Veggie Lovers'		
hand-tossed, medium pie	1 slice	222

Prot. MGS	Carbs. GMS	Sodium MGS	Fiber GMS	Fat GMS	Sat. Fat GMS	Chol. MGS	% Fat Cal.
20.0	28.0	738	2.0	10.0	3.0	25	36%
8.0	26.0	618	2.0	18.0	3.0	25	58%
37.0	76.0	1335	8.0	29.0	12.5	53	39%
31.0	68.0	na	na	18.0	na	na	29%
12.0	20.0	678	2.0	11.0	3.0	27	43%
23.0	45.0	na	na	17.0	na	na	36%
10.0	25.0	1208	2.0	9.0	4.0	21	38%
19.0	28.0	981	3.0	16.0	4.0	43	43%
14.0	27.0	861	3.0	25.0	5.0	34	62%
18.0	20.0	949	2.0	19.0	4.0	46	53%
15.0	28.0	803	3.0	11.0	3.0	25	37%
10.0	27.0	683	3.0	19.0	3.0	25	58%
36.0	71.0	na	na	23.0	na	na	32%
13.0	20.0	713	2.0	12.0	3.0	25	45%
27.0	51.0	na	na	23.0	na	na	40%
29.0	44.0	1336	5.0	21.0	10.3	56	41%
17.0	28.0	980	3.0	10.0	3.0	32	33%
12.0	27.0	860	3.0	19.0	4.0	32	57%
16.0	20.0	700	2.0	12.0	3.0	35	43%
17.0	28.0	894	3.0	12.0	3.0	29	37%
16.0	27.0	774	3.0	16.0	3.0	29	46%
33.0	76.0	1313	9.0	28.0	11.2	49	39%
36.0	74.0	na	na	22.0	na	na	31%
15.0	20.0	819	3.0	14.0	3.0	31	48%
27.0	51.0	na	na	21.0	na	na	37%
13.0	28.0	641	3.0	7.0	3.0	17	28%

Food Name	Serving Size	Total Calories
'Pan Pizza'	1 slice	249
'Thin 'n Crispy' medium pie	1 slice	192

PONDEROSA

Food Name	Serving Size	Total Calories
ALFALFA SPROUTS	1 oz	10
APPLE		
canned	4 oz	90
rings, spiced	4 oz	100
whole, raw	1 med	80
APPLESAUCE	4 oz	80
BANANA		
chips	.2 oz	25
whole, raw	1 med	87
BARBECUE SAUCE	1 tbsp	25
BEAN SPROUTS	1 oz	10
BEANS		
baked	4 oz	170
garbanzo	1 oz	102
green	3.5 oz	20
BEETS, diced	4 oz	55
BREADSTICKS		
Italian	1 breadstick	100
sesame	2 breadsticks	35
BROCCOLI, raw	1 oz	9
CABBAGE		
green, raw	1 oz	9
red, raw	1 oz	1
CANTALOUPE	1 wedge	13
CARAMEL TOPPING	1 oz	100
CARROTS		
raw	3.5 oz	31
raw	1 oz	12

Prot. MGS	Carbs. GMS	Sodium MGS	Fiber GMS	Fat GMS	Sat. Fat GMS	Chol. MGS	% Fat Cal.
7.0	27.0	521	3.0	15.0	3.0	17	54%
11.0	20.0	551	3.0	8.0	3.0	17	38%
1.0	1.0	0	(mq)	0.0	0.0	0	0%
0.0	22.0	15	(mq)	0.0	0.0	0	0%
0.0	24.0	20	(mq)	0.0	0.0	0	0%
0.0	20.0	1	(mq)	1.0	na	0	11%
0.0	20.0	20	(mq)	0.0	0.0	0	0%
0.2	3.3	tr	(mq)	1.3	na	0	47%
1.1	22.6	1	(mq)	0.2	(tr)	0	2%
0.0	5.0	260	na	0.0	0.0	0	0%
1.1	1.9	1	(mq)	tr	0.0	0	0%
6.0	21.0	330	(mq)	6.0	(mq)	0	32%
6.0	17.0	7	na	0.0	na	0	0%
1.0	3.0	391	na	0.0	na	0	0%
0.4	12.5	307	(mq)	0.4	na	0	7%
4.0	19.0	200	(mq)	1.0	na	0	9%
1.0	6.0	60	na	0.0	na	0	0%
1.0	1.7	4	(mq)	0.9	na	0	90%
1.0	1.9	7	(mq)	0.0	0.0	0	0%
0.1	0.3	1	(mq)	0.0	0.0	0	0%
0.3	3.3	5	(mq)	0.0	0.0	0	0%
0.4	26.2	72	na	0.7	na	2	6%
1.0	7.0	33	na	0.0	na	0	0%
0.3	2.8	13	(mq)	0.1	(tr)	0	8%

Food Name	Serving Size	Total Calories
CAULIFLOWER		
breaded	4 oz	115
raw	1 oz	8
CELERY, raw	1 oz	4
CHEESE, imitation, shredded	1 oz	90
CHEESE SAUCE	2 oz	52
CHEESE SPREAD	1 oz	98
CHEESE TOPPING, herb and garlic	1 tbsp	100
CHICKEN		
breast	5.5 oz	98
wing	2 pieces	213
CHOCOLATE TOPPING	1 oz	89
CHOPPED STEAK		
5.3-oz size	1 serving	296
4-oz size	1 serving	225
CHOW MEIN NOODLES	.2 oz	25
COCKTAIL SAUCE	1 oz	34
COCONUT, shredded	.2 oz	25
COFFEE	6 oz	2
COOKIE, vanilla wafer	2 wafers	35
CORN	3.5 oz	90
COTTAGE CHEESE	4 oz	120
CRACKER		
Melba snacks	2 crackers	18
'Ritz'	2 crackers	40
sesame, 'Meal Mate'	2 crackers	45
CROUTONS	1 oz	115
CUCUMBER, raw	1 oz	4
EGG, boiled, diced	2 oz	93
FISH. See also individual listings.		
baked, 'Bake 'R Broil'	5.2 oz	230
fried	3.2 oz	190
nugget	1 nugget	31

Prot. MGS	Carbs. GMS	Sodium MGS	Fiber GMS	Fat GMS	Sat. Fat GMS	Chol. MGS	% Fat Cal.
4.0	23.0	446	na	1.0	na	1	8%
0.8	1.5	4	(mq)	0.1	(tr)	0	11%
0.3	1.1	36	(mq)	0.0	0.0	0	0%
6.0	1.0	420	na	7.0	na	5	70%
1.2	6.4	355	na	2.0	(mq)	4	35%
4.0	4.0	188	na	7.0	na	26	64%
0.0	0.0	120	na	10.0	na	0	90%
20.0	1.0	400	na	2.0	na	54	18%
11.0	11.0	610	na	9.0	na	75	38%
0.5	24.3	37	na	0.3	na	0	3%
25.0	1.0	296	na	22.0	na	105	67%
19.0	1.0	150	na	16.0	na	80	64%
0.6	3.0	42	(mq)	1.2	na	0	43%
0.4	6.2	453	na	1.0	na	0	26%
0.2	2.0	14	(mq)	1.9	(mq)	0	68%
0.0	0.5	26	0	0.0	0.0	0	0%
0.0	6.0	25	na	1.0	na	5	26%
3.0	21.0	5	(mq)	0.4	na	0	4%
15.0	5.0	330	na	5.0	na	17	38%
1.0	4.0	60	(mq)	0.0	0.0	0	0%
0.0	4.0	50	na	2.0	na	0	45%
1.0	6.0	95	na	2.0	na	0	40%
4.0	18.0	351	na	4.0	na	0	31%
0.3	1.0	2	(mq)	0.0	0.0	0	0%
7.0	1.0	74	na	7.0	na	260	68%
19.0	10.0	330	na	13.0	na	50	51%
9.0	17.0	170	na	9.0	na	15	43%
1.7	1.9	52	(mq)	1.7	(mq)	8	49%

Food Name	Serving Size	Total Calories
FRENCH FRIES	3 oz	120
FRUIT COCKTAIL	4 oz	97
GELATIN DESSERT, plain	4 oz	71
GRANOLA	.2 oz	24
GRAPES	10 grapes	34
GRAVY		
brown	2 oz	25
turkey	2 oz	25
HALIBUT, broiled	6 oz	170
HAM, diced	2 oz	120
HONEYDEW MELON	1 wedge	25
HOT DOG	1.6 oz	144
ICE MILK		
chocolate	3.5 oz	152
vanilla	3.5 oz	150
ICED TEA	6 oz	2
LEMON	1 wedge	3
LETTUCE	1 oz	5
MACARONI AND CHEESE	1 oz	17
MARGARINE		
liquid	1 tbsp	100
whipped	1 tbsp	34
MEATBALLS	2 pieces	115
MILK		
chocolate	8 oz	208
whole	8 oz	159
MOUSSE		
chocolate	4 oz	312
chocolate	1 oz	78
strawberry	4 oz	297
strawberry	1 oz	74
MUSHROOMS, raw	1 oz	8
OKRA, breaded	4 oz	124

Prot. MGS	Carbs. GMS	Sodium MGS	Fiber GMS	Fat GMS	Sat. Fat GMS	Chol. MGS	% Fat Cal.
2.0	17.0	39	na	4.0	na	3	30%
0.5	25.1	7	(mq)	0.2	(tr)	0	2%
1.0	17.0	73	na	0.0	na	0	0%
0.6	3.1	na	(mq)	1.0	na	0	38%
0.3	8.7	2	(mq)	0.2	(tr)	0	5%
0.6	3.9	167	na	1.0	na	0	36%
0.7	5.1	228	na	0.2	na	0	7%
35.0	0.0	68	0	2.4	(mq)	(mq)	13%
9.0	1.0	780	na	10.0	na	76	75%
0.6	5.8	9	(mq)	0.2	(tr)	0	7%
5.0	1.0	460	na	13.0	na	27	81%
4.0	30.0	70	na	3.0	na	22	18%
4.0	30.0	58	na	3.0	na	20	18%
0.1	0.5	0	0	0.0	0.0	0	0%
0.1	0.8	0	(mq)	0.1	(tr)	0	30%
0.0	2.0	5	na	0.0	na	0	0%
0.7	4.4	80	(mq)	0.5	na	1	26%
0.0	0.0	110	0	11.0	(mq)	0	99%
0.0	0.0	65	0	1.2	(mq)	0	32%
5.0	2.0	16	na	4.0	na	21	31%
7.9	25.9	149	0	8.5	(mq)	33	37%
8.5	12.0	122	0	8.6	(mq)	34	49%
0.0	28.0	72	na	18.0	na	0	52%
0.0	6.9	18	na	4.4	(mq)	0	51%
0.0	25.0	68	na	18.0	na	0	55%
0.0	6.3	17	na	4.6	(mq)	0	56%
0.8	1.3	4	(mq)	0.1	(tr)	0	11%
3.0	23.0	483	na	1.0	na	1	7%

Food Name	Serving Size	Total Calories
OLIVES		
black	1 piece	4
green	1 piece	4
ONION		
green, raw	1 piece	7
red, raw	1 oz	11
yellow, raw	1 oz	11
ONION RINGS, breaded	4 oz	213
ORANGE	1 piece	45
ORANGE ROUGHY, broiled	5 oz	139
PASTA. See also individual listings.		
	2 oz	78
PEACH, canned	4 oz	70
PEANUT TOPPING, granulated	.2 oz	30
PEAR, canned	4 oz	98
PEAS	3.5 oz	67
PEPPER, CHERRY, raw	2 pieces	7
PEPPER, GREEN, raw	1 oz	6
PICKLE		
dill, spear	.14 oz	1
sweet, chips	.14 oz	4
PINEAPPLE		
fresh	1 wedge	11
tidbits	4 oz	95
PORTERHOUSE STEAK		
choice	16 oz	640
non-graded	13 oz	440
POTATO, BAKED	7.2 oz	145
POTATO WEDGES	3.5 oz	130
POTATOES, MASHED	4 oz	62
PUDDING		
banana	4 oz	207
banana	1 oz	52

Prot. MGS	Carbs. GMS	Sodium MGS	Fiber GMS	Fat GMS	Sat. Fat GMS	Chol. MGS	% Fat Cal.
0.0	0.1	24	(mq)	0.4	na	0	90%
0.0	0.0	69	(mq)	0.4	na	0	90%
0.2	1.6	1	(mq)	0.1	(tr)	0	13%
0.4	2.5	3	(mq)	0.0	0.0	0	0%
0.4	2.5	3	(mq)	0.0	0.0	0	0%
3.0	30.0	620	na	9.0	na	2	38%
1.2	11.3	1	(mq)	0.1	(tr)	0	2%
tr	21.0	88	na	5.0	na	28	32%
2.4	16.1	1	(mq)	0.3	na	0	3%
0.0	18.0	10	(mq)	0.0	0.0	0	0%
1.2	1.1	0	(mq)	2.3	(mq)	0	69%
0.5	25.0	7	(mq)	0.5	na	0	5%
5.0	12.0	120	na	0.0	na	0	0%
0.2	1.4	415	(mq)	0.2	(tr)	0	26%
0.3	1.4	4	(mq)	0.1	(tr)	0	15%
0.0	0.1	54	(mq)	0.0	0.0	0	0%
0.1	1.0	1	(mq)	0.0	0.0	0	0%
0.1	2.9	tr	(mq)	0.1	(tr)	0	8%
0.4	24.8	2	(mq)	0.2	na	0	2%
57.0	3.0	1130	na	31.0	na	82	44%
43.0	1.0	1844	na	30.0	na	67	61%
4.0	33.0	6	na	0.0	na	0	0%
3.0	16.0	170	na	6.0	na	na	42%
2.0	13.0	191	na	0.0	na	20	0%
1.0	27.0	114	na	10.0	na	0	43%
0.4	6.4	29	na	2.4	(mq)	0	42%

Food Name	Serving Size	Total Calories
RADISH, raw	1 oz	4
RIB EYE STEAK		
choice	6 oz	282
non-graded	5 oz	219
RICE PILAF	4 oz	160
ROLL		
dinner	1 piece	184
sourdough	1 piece	110
SALAD		
chicken	3.5 oz	212
chicken macaroni	3.5 oz	335
macaroni	3.5 oz	335
pasta	3.5 oz	268
potato	3.5 oz	126
turkey-ham	3.5 oz	186
SALAD DRESSING		
blue cheese	1 oz	130
coleslaw	1 oz	150
creamy Italian	1 oz	103
cucumber, reduced calorie	1 oz	69
Italian, reduced calorie	1 oz	31
Parmesan pepper	1 oz	150
ranch	1 oz	147
salad oil	1 tbsp	120
sweet and tangy	1 oz	122
Thousand Island	1 oz	113
SALMON, broiled	6 oz	192
SCROD, baked	7 oz	120
SHRIMP		
fried	7 pieces	230
mini	6 pieces	47
SIRLOIN STEAK, choice	7 oz	241
SOUR CREAM	1 tbsp	26

Prot. MGS	Carbs. GMS	Sodium MGS	Fiber GMS	Fat GMS	Sat. Fat GMS	Chol. MGS	% Fat Cal.
0.3	0.9	5	(mq)	0.0	0.0	0	0%
29.0	1.0	570	na	14.0	na	60	45%
25.0	1.0	1130	na	13.0	na	75	53%
4.0	26.0	450	na	4.0	na	22	23%
5.0	33.0	311	na	3.0	na	0	15%
4.0	22.0	230	(mq)	1.0	na	0	8%
11.0	8.0	334	na	15.0	na	42	64%
8.0	49.0	431	na	12.0	na	9	32%
7.6	49.2	431	(mq)	11.7	(mq)	9	31%
6.0	34.0	441	na	12.0	na	0	40%
2.0	16.0	300	na	6.0	na	7	43%
7.5	10.1	655	na	12.8	(mq)	12	62%
1.0	1.0	266	na	14.0	na	27	97%
tr	6.0	284	na	14.0	na	31	84%
0.0	3.0	373	na	10.0	na	0	87%
tr	3.0	315	na	6.0	na	0	78%
0.0	1.0	371	na	3.0	na	0	87%
1.0	2.0	281	na	15.0	na	9	90%
tr	1.0	297	na	15.0	na	3	92%
0.0	0.0	0	0	13.3	(mq)	0	100%
tr	8.0	347	na	10.0	na	1	74%
tr	8.0	405	na	10.0	na	9	80%
37.0	3.0	72	na	3.0	na	60	14%
27.0	0.0	80	na	1.0	na	65	8%
22.0	31.0	612	na	1.0	na	105	4%
5.0	6.0	125	na	1.0	na	22	19%
35.0	1.0	570	na	11.0	na	63	41%
0.4	0.5	6	0	2.5	(mq)	5	87%

Food Name	Serving Size	Total Calories
SPAGHETTI, w/sauce	6 oz	188
SPAGHETTI ENTRÉE	2 oz	78
SPAGHETTI SAUCE	4 oz	110
SPINACH, raw	1 oz	7
STEAK ENTRÉE. See individual listings.		
STEAK KABOBS, meat only	3 oz	153
STEAK SANDWICH	4 oz	208
STRAWBERRIES	2 oz	14
STRAWBERRY GLAZE	1 oz	37
STRAWBERRY TOPPING	1 oz	71
STUFFING	4 oz	230
SWEET AND SOUR SAUCE	1 oz	37
SWORDFISH, broiled	5.9 oz	271
T-BONE STEAK		
choice	10 oz	444
non-graded	8 oz	178
TARTAR SAUCE	1 oz	85
TERIYAKI STEAK	5 oz	174
TOMATO	1 oz	6
TORTILLA CHIPS	1 oz	150
TROUT, broiled	5 oz	228
TURKEY, julienne	1 oz	29
WATERMELON	1 wedge	111
WHIPPED TOPPING	1 oz	80
YOGURT, FROZEN		
fruit	4 oz	115
vanilla	4 oz	110
ZUCCHINI		
breaded	4 oz	102
raw	1 oz	5

Prot. MGS	Carbs. GMS	Sodium MGS	Fiber GMS	Fat GMS	Sat. Fat GMS	Chol. MGS	% Fat Cal.
5.0	33.0	520	na	5.0	na	0	24%
2.4	16.1	1	(mq)	0.3	na	0	3%
2.0	17.0	520	na	4.0	(mq)	0	33%
0.9	1.2	20	(mq)	0.1	(tr)	0	13%
26.0	2.0	280	na	5.0	na	67	29%
20.0	2.0	850	na	11.0	na	62	48%
0.3	3.1	61	(mq)	0.2	(tr)	tr	13%
0.0	9.5	4	na	0.0	0.0	0	0%
0.1	23.6	29	na	0.2	na	0	3%
6.0	27.0	800	na	11.0	na	22	43%
na	8.0	80	na	na	na	0	0%
44.0	0.0	0	na	10.0	na	84	33%
44.0	2.0	850	na	18.0	na	80	36%
24.7	1.6	850	0	8.5	(mq)	71	43%
0.1	11.1	477	na	9.3	(mq)	9	98%
32.0	5.0	1420	na	3.0	na	64	16%
0.3	1.3	1	(mq)	0.1	(tr)	0	15%
3.0	16.0	80	(mq)	8.0	(mq)	0	48%
30.0	1.0	51	na	4.0	na	110	16%
5.0	1.0	192	na	1.0	na	15	31%
2.1	27.3	4	(mq)	0.9	na	0	7%
0.0	5.0	16	na	7.0	na	0	79%
5.0	23.0	70	na	1.0	na	5	8%
5.0	18.0	75	0	2.0	na	6	16%
3.0	18.0	584	na	1.0	na	1	9%
0.3	1.0	tr	(mq)	0.0	0.0	0	0%

Food Name	Serving Size	Total Calories

POPEYES

APPLE PIE	3.1 oz	290
BISCUIT	2.3 oz	250
CHICKEN		
breast, mild	3.7 oz	270
breast, spicy	3.7 oz	270
leg, mild	1.7 oz	120
leg, spicy	1.7 oz	120
nugget	4.2 oz	410
thigh, mild	3.1 oz	300
thigh, spicy	3.1 oz	300
wing, mild	1.6 oz	160
wing, spicy	1.6 oz	160
COLESLAW	4 oz	149
CORN, on the cob	5.2 oz	90
FRENCH FRIES	3 oz	240
ONION RINGS	3.1 oz	310
RED BEANS AND RICE	5.9 oz	270

QUINCY'S

BEANS, green, 4.3 oz	1 serving	40
BROCCOLI, cream of, 9.2 oz	1 serving	193
CATFISH FILLET, 2 pieces, 6.9 oz	1 serving	309
CHEESEBURGER, 1/4-lb patty	1 serving	451
CHICKEN, breast, grilled, 5 oz	1 serving	145
CHICKEN STRIPS, 4 pieces, 4.5 oz	1 serving	318
CHILI, w/beans, 9.2 oz	1 serving	346
CHOPPED STEAK		
5.8-oz size	1 serving	466
luncheon, 4-oz size	1 serving	350
CHOWDER, clam, 9.2 oz	1 serving	198

Prot. MGS	Carbs. GMS	Sodium MGS	Fiber GMS	Fat GMS	Sat. Fat GMS	Chol. MGS	% Fat Cal.
2.5	36.6	820	2.0	15.8	na	10	49%
3.7	26.1	430	1.0	14.9	na	<5	54%
23.1	9.2	660	2.0	15.9	na	60	53%
23.1	9.2	590	2.0	15.9	na	60	53%
10.3	4.4	240	0	7.3	na	40	55%
10.3	4.4	240	0	7.3	na	40	55%
17.1	17.9	660	3.0	31.9	na	55	70%
14.7	9.3	620	<1.0	22.7	na	70	68%
14.7	9.3	450	<1.0	22.7	na	70	68%
9.3	6.6	290	0	10.7	na	40	60%
9.3	6.6	290	0	10.7	na	40	60%
0.9	13.6	271	3.0	11.2	na	3	68%
4.0	21.4	20	9.0	2.9	na	0	29%
3.5	30.8	610	3.0	12.2	na	10	46%
4.9	31.1	210	2.0	19.3	na	25	56%
7.5	29.7	680	7.0	16.9	na	10	56%
2.0	7.0	500	(mq)	1.0	na	0	23%
3.0	13.0	1045	(mq)	14.0	(mq)	na	65%
26.0	19.0	101	(mq)	12.0	(mq)	(mq)	35%
28.0	32.0	432	(mq)	23.0	(mq)	(mq)	46%
35.0	0.0	140	0	0.4	(mq)	72	2%
39.0	4.0	(mq)	(mq)	15.0	(mq)	(mq)	42%
20.0	32.0	1380	(mq)	16.0	(mq)	(mq)	42%
40.0	0.0	96	0	34.0	(mq)	(mq)	66%
30.0	0.0	72	0	25.0	(mq)	(mq)	64%
6.0	15.0	1185	(mq)	14.0	(mq)	(mq)	64%

Food Name	Serving Size	Total Calories
COLESLAW, 2.1 oz	1 serving	60
CORNBREAD, 1.9 oz	1 serving	178
FRENCH FRIES, steak fries, 5.5 oz	1 serving	426
HAMBURGER, 1/4-lb patty	1 serving	403
MARGARINE, 1 oz	1 serving	204
MUSHROOM SAUCE, 3 oz	1 serving	27
PEPPERS AND ONIONS, 4 oz	1 serving	80
POTATO, BAKED, w/o butter, 8.8 oz	1 serving	181
POTATOES, MASHED, w/gravy, 3.8 oz	1 serving	100
RIB EYE STEAK, 7.3 oz	1 serving	665
RICE, Cajun, 3.9 oz	1 serving	150
SHRIMP		
7 pieces, 3.9 oz	1 serving	248
2.8 oz	1 serving	250
SIRLOIN STEAK		
large, 7.7 oz	1 serving	852
petite, 4 oz	1 serving	446
regular, 5.9 oz	1 serving	649
sirloin club, 4.8 oz	1 serving	283
sirloin tips, 4 oz	1 serving	236
STEAK. See also individual listings.		
country style, w/mushroom sauce, 6 oz	1 serving	288
STEAK FILLET, 5.6 oz	1 serving	331
T-BONE STEAK, 7.8 oz	1 serving	1045
VEGETABLE BEEF SOUP, 8.6 oz	1 serving	78

RALLY'S

CHEESEBURGER

'Bacon Cheeseburger'	1 sandwich	622
'Double Cheeseburger'	1 sandwich	733
'Rallyburger' w/cheese	1 sandwich	486

Prot. MGS	Carbs. GMS	Sodium MGS	Fiber GMS	Fat GMS	Sat. Fat GMS	Chol. MGS	% Fat Cal.
<1.0	4.0	75	(mq)	5.0	(mq)	na	75%
4.0	28.0	263	(mq)	6.0	(mq)	na	30%
7.0	56.0	90	(mq)	21.0	(mq)	na	44%
25.0	32.0	284	(mq)	19.0	(mq)	(mq)	42%
<1.0	<1.0	268	0	22.0	(mq)	0	97%
1.0	5.0	366	na	<1.0	na	na	0%
1.0	8.0	11	(mq)	5.0	(mq)	na	56%
5.0	41.0	8	(mq)	<1.0	na	0	0%
5.0	10.5	460	3.0	6.0	na	<5	54%
31.0	0.0	205	0	60.0	(mq)	(mq)	81%
10.0	17.4	1260	3.0	5.4	na	25	32%
22.0	11.0	205	(mq)	12.0	(mq)	(mq)	44%
15.6	13.2	650	3.0	16.4	na	110	59%
50.0	0.0	241	0	70.0	(mq)	(mq)	74%
26.0	0.0	118	0	37.0	(mq)	(mq)	75%
38.0	0.0	206	0	54.0	(mq)	(mq)	75%
44.0	0.0	160	0	10.0	(mq)	(mq)	32%
37.0	0.0	113	0	9.0	(mq)	(mq)	34%
18.0	17.0	315	(mq)	19.0	(mq)	(mq)	59%
51.0	0.0	159	0	12.0	(mq)	(mq)	33%
43.0	0.0	222	0	95.0	(mq)	(mq)	82%
5.0	10.0	1045	(mq)	2.0	(mq)	(mq)	23%
33.0	34.5	1629	na	40.3	na	99	58%
42.4	33.9	1473	na	49.1	na	92	60%
24.2	33.4	1185	na	29.4	na	79	54%

Food Name	Serving Size	Total Calories
CHEESEBURGER MEAL		
'Large Combo' w/soft drink	1 meal	1018
'Small Combo'w/soft drink	1 meal	764
CHICKEN SANDWICH	1 sandwich	531
CHILI	8 oz	340
FRENCH FRIES		
large order	1 serving	317
regular order	1 serving	158
HAMBURGER, 'Rallyburger'	1 sandwich	436
HAMBURGER MEAL		
'Large Combo' w/ soft drink	1 meal	968
'Small Combo' w/soft drink	1 meal	714
ICED TEA		
16-oz size	1 serving	3
32-oz size	1 serving	6
MILKSHAKE		
chocolate	1 serving	411
strawberry banana	1 serving	399
vanilla	1 serving	320
SAUSAGE		
'Smokin' Sausage'	1 serving	724
'Smokin' Sausage' w/chili	1 serving	830
SOFT DRINK		
Coca-Cola, 32-oz size	1 serving	216
Coca-Cola, 16-oz size	1 serving	120
Diet Coke, 32-oz size	1 serving	1
Diet Coke, 16-oz size	1 serving	1
Dr. Pepper, 32-oz size	1 serving	216
Dr. Pepper, 16-oz size	1 serving	120
Fanta Orange, 32-oz size	1 serving	264
Fanta Orange, 16-oz size	1 serving	147
Fanta Root Beer, 32-oz size	1 serving	234
Fanta Root Beer, 16-oz size	1 serving	130

Prot. MGS	Carbs. GMS	Sodium MGS	Fiber GMS	Fat GMS	Sat. Fat GMS	Chol. MGS	% Fat Cal.
29.3	129.4	1645	na	45.0	na	89	40%
32.6	84.7	1416	na	37.2	na	84	44%
18.1	39.5	364	na	30.8	na	18	52%
22.2	21.3	1199	na	19.0	na	67	50%
5.1	39.0	439	na	15.6	na	10	44%
2.5	19.5	219	na	7.8	na	5	44%
21.2	32.9	955	na	24.9	na	67	51%
26.3	128.9	1415	na	40.5	na	76	38%
23.8	84.1	1186	na	32.7	na	71	41%
0.0	0.0	0	0	0.0	0.0	0	0%
0.0	0.0	0	0	0.0	0.0	0	0%
9.7	72.5	262	na	11.8	na	38	26%
9.4	69.5	223	na	11.3	na	38	25%
9.4	49.0	197	na	11.3	na	38	32%
28.0	31.0	1998	na	55.0	na	40	68%
34.8	35.0	2163	na	62.0	na	67	67%
0.0	57.0	21	0	0.0	0.0	0	0%
0.0	32.0	12	0	0.0	0.0	0	0%
0.0	0.5	39	0	0.0	0.0	0	0%
0.0	0.3	22	0	0.0	0.0	0	0%
0.0	57.0	27	0	0.0	0.0	0	0%
0.0	32.0	15	0	0.0	0.0	0	0%
0.0	69.0	21	0	0.0	0.0	0	0%
0.0	38.4	12	0	0.0	0.0	0	0%
0.0	60.0	30	0	0.0	0.0	0	0%
0.0	33.0	17	0	0.0	0.0	0	0%

Food Name	Serving Size	Total Calories
Ramblin' Root Beer, 32-oz size	1 serving	264
Ramblin' Root Beer, 16-oz size	1 serving	147
Sprite, 32-oz size	1 serving	213
Sprite, 16-oz size	1 serving	119
TACO, soft	1 taco	223

RAX

Food Name	Serving Size	Total Calories
ALFALFA SPROUTS	1 oz	8
ALFREDO SAUCE	3.5 oz	80
APPLESAUCE	1 cup	100
BACON BITS	.5 oz	40
BARBECUE MEAT TOPPING	3.25 oz	140
BARBECUE SANDWICH, 5.7 oz	1 serving	420
BARBECUE SAUCE	.5 oz	11
BEANS		
garbanzo	1/2 cup	360
kidney	1 cup	220
BEEF SANDWICH		
'BBC' beef, bacon, chicken, 8 oz	1 serving	720
Philly beef and cheese, 8.25 oz	1 serving	480
BEETS	1 cup	60
BREADSTICK, sesame	1 oz	150
BROCCOLI, raw	1/2 cup	16
BROCCOLI SOUP, cream of	3.5 oz	50
CABBAGE		
green, raw	1 cup	16
red, raw	1/4 cup	4
CANTALOUPE	2 pieces	16
CARROT, raw	1/4 cup	8
CATSUP	1 tbsp	6
CAULIFLOWER, raw	1/2 cup	16
CELERY, raw	1 tbsp	1

Prot. MGS	Carbs. GMS	Sodium MGS	Fiber GMS	Fat GMS	Sat. Fat GMS	Chol. MGS	% Fat Cal.
0.0	69.0	30	0	0.0	0.0	0	0%
0.0	38.4	17	0	0.0	0.0	0	0%
0.0	54.0	69	0	0.0	0.0	0	0%
0.0	30.0	12	0	0.0	0.0	0	0%
12.1	17.0	377	na	9.9	na	36	40%
<1.0	2.0	<1	(mq)	<1.0	(tr)	0	0%
2.0	12.0	70	(mq)	3.0	(mq)	10	34%
<1.0	26.0	5	(mq)	<1.0	(tr)	0	0%
5.0	<1.0	427	0	2.0	(mq)	12	45%
13.0	13.0	898	na	4.0	(mq)	24	26%
21.0	53.0	1343	(mq)	14.0	(mq)	24	30%
0.0	3.0	158	na	0.0	0.0	0	0%
20.0	60.0	26	(mq)	5.0	(mq)	0	13%
14.0	40.0	8	(mq)	1.0	(mq)	0	4%
30.0	40.0	1873	(mq)	49.0	(mq)	137	61%
25.0	44.0	1346	(mq)	22.0	(mq)	49	41%
2.0	12.0	73	(mq)	<1.0	(tr)	0	0%
3.0	13.0	405	(mq)	10.0	(mq)	0	60%
2.0	2.0	7	(mq)	<1.0	(tr)	0	0%
1.0	6.0	219	(mq)	2.0	(mq)	<1	36%
<1.0	4.0	18	(mq)	<1.0	(tr)	0	0%
<1.0	<1.0	6	(mq)	<1.0	(tr)	0	0%
<1.0	4.0	6	(mq)	<1.0	(tr)	0	0%
<1.0	2.0	<1	(mq)	<1.0	(tr)	0	0%
<1.0	2.0	50	(mq)	<1.0	(tr)	0	0%
<.0	2.0	6	(mq)	<1.0	(tr)	0	0%
<1.0	<1.0	10	(mq)	<1.0	(tr)	0	0%

Food Name	Serving Size	Total Calories
CHEESE		
cheddar, imitation, shredded	1 oz	90
cheddar, tidbits	1 oz	160
Parmesan, substitute	1 oz	80
CHEESE SAUCE		
nacho	3.5 oz	470
regular	3.5 oz	420
CHICKEN NOODLE SOUP	3.5 oz	40
CHILI TOPPING	3 oz	80
CHOW MEIN NOODLES	1 oz	140
COCONUT	1 oz	160
COLESLAW	3.5 oz	70
COOKIE, chocolate chip	1 cookie	130
COTTAGE CHEESE	1 cup	250
CRACKER, 'Saltines'	2 crackers	16
CROUTONS	.5 oz	40
CUCUMBER	2 slices	2
EGG, boiled, salad topping	1.5 oz	70
FISH SANDWICH, 7 oz	1 serving	460
FRENCH FRIES		
large order, 4.5 oz	1 serving	390
large order, unsalted, 4.5 oz	1 serving	390
regular order, 3 oz	1 serving	260
regular order, unsalted, 3 oz	1 serving	260
GELATIN		
lime	1/2 cup	90
strawberry	1/2 cup	90
GRAPEFRUIT, sections	1 cup	80
GRAPE	1 cup	100
HAM AND CHEESE SANDWICH,		
w/Swiss cheese, 7.9 oz	1 serving	430
HONEYDEW MELON	2 pieces	25
HOT CHOCOLATE	6 oz	110

Prot. MGS	Carbs. GMS	Sodium MGS	Fiber GMS	Fat GMS	Sat. Fat GMS	Chol. MGS	% Fat Cal.
6.0	2.0	310	na	6.0	(mq)	6	60%
3.0	12.0	445	0	11.0	(mq)	<1	62%
8.0	2.0	1000	(mq)	4.0	(mq)	<1	45%
10.0	57.0	190	na	22.0	na	11	42%
10.0	58.0	365	na	17.0	na	11	36%
2.0	8.0	1040	(mq)	<1.0	(mq)	10	0%
8.0	8.0	221	(mq)	2.0	(mq)	18	23%
4.0	17.0	242	(mq)	6.0	(mq)	<1	39%
<1.0	15.0	<1	(mq)	11.0	(mq)	0	62%
1.0	8.0	187	(mq)	4.0	(mq)	<1	51%
1.0	17.0	65	(mq)	6.0	(mq)	<1	42%
33.0	7.0	561	(mq)	10.0	(mq)	47	36%
<1.0	4.0	70	(mq)	<1.0	(mq)	<1	0%
2.0	8.0	155	(mq)	<1.0	(mq)	<1	0%
<1.0	<1.0	<1	(mq)	<1.0	(tr)	0	0%
6.0	<1.0	32	0	5.0	(mq)	267	64%
14.0	58.0	935	(mq)	17.0	(mq)	<1	33%
3.0	50.0	104	(mq)	20.0	(mq)	16	46%
3.0	50.0	66	(mq)	20.0	(mq)	16	46%
2.0	33.0	69	(mq)	13.0	(mq)	10	45%
2.0	33.0	44	(mq)	13.0	(mq)	10	45%
2.0	20.0	90	0	<1.0	(tr)	0	0%
2.0	20.0	90	0	<1.0	(tr)	0	0%
2.0	18.0	10	(mq)	<1.0	(tr)	0	0%
<1.0	25.0	5	(mq)	<1.0	(tr)	0	0%
23.0	42.0	1737	(mq)	23.0	(mq)	37	48%
<1.0	6.0	5	(mq)	<1.0	(tr)	0	0%
2.0	<1.0	120	(mq)	11.0	(mq)	<1	90%

Food Name	Serving Size	Total Calories
KALE	1 oz	16
LETTUCE	1 leaf	2
MARGARINE, liquid	1 tbsp	100
MILKSHAKE		
chocolate, w/o whipped topping	1 serving	560
strawberry, w/o whipped topping	1 serving	560
vanilla, w/o whipped topping	1 serving	500
MUSHROOM SAUCE	1 oz	16
MUSHROOMS, raw	1/4 cup	4
OLIVES	3.5 oz	110
ONION		
diced	.5 oz	10
green	1/4 cup	10
raw	1/4 cup	12
PASTA AND NOODLES. See also individual listings.		
pasta shells	3.5 oz	170
pasta/vegetable blend	3.5 oz	100
rainbow rotini	3.5 oz	180
PEACH	2 slices	16
PEAS	1 oz	25
PEPPER, BANANA, rings	1 tbsp	2
PEPPER, CHERRY	1 tbsp	6
PEPPER, GREEN	1/4 cup	8
PEPPER, JALAPEÑO	1 oz	6
PICKLE	1 spear	8
PINEAPPLE		
canned	3.5 oz	100
fresh	3-oz slice	45
POTATO, BAKED		
barbecue, w/2 oz cheese	1 serving	730
chili, w/2 oz cheese	1 serving	700
plain, 8.8 oz	1 serving	270
plain, w/margarine, 9.3 oz	1 serving	370

Prot. MGS	Carbs. GMS	Sodium MGS	Fiber GMS	Fat GMS	Sat. Fat GMS	Chol. MGS	% Fat Cal.
2.0	2.0	21	(mq)	<1.0	(tr)	0	0%
0.0	0.0	<1	(mq)	0.0	(tr)	0	0%
<1.0	<1.0	100	0	11.0	(mq)	0	99%
13.0	97.0	239	(tr)	13.0	(mq)	63	21%
13.0	97.0	226	(tr)	13.0	(mq)	62	21%
13.0	81.0	286	0	14.0	(mq)	58	25%
1.0	1.0	113	na	<1.0	0.0	0	0%
<1.0	<1.0	<1	(mq)	<1.0	(tr)	0	0%
<1.0	6.0	880	(mq)	10.0	(mq)	0	82%
<1.0	1.0	1	(mq)	<1.0	(tr)	0	0%
<1.0	2.0	1	(mq)	<1.0	(tr)	0	0%
<1.0	3.0	3	(mq)	<1.0	(tr)	0	0%
7.0	27.0	2	(mq)	4.0	(mq)	0	21%
4.0	12.0	11	(mq)	4.0	(mq)	0	36%
6.0	30.0	9	(mq)	4.0	(mq)	2	20%
<1.0	4.0	<1	(mq)	<1.0	(tr)	0	0%
2.0	4.0	35	(mq)	<1.0	(tr)	0	0%
<1.0	<1.0	20	(mq)	<1.0	(tr)	0	0%
<1.0	<1.0	180	(mq)	<1.0	(tr)	0	0%
<1.0	1.0	5	(mq)	<1.0	(tr)	0	0%
<1.0	1.0	231	(mq)	<1.0	(tr)	0	0%
<1.0	2.0	928	(mq)	<1.0	(tr)	0	0%
<1.0	25.0	10	(mq)	<1.0	(tr)	0	0%
<1.0	12.0	1	(mq)	<1.0	(tr)	0	0%
24.0	104.0	1071	(mq)	24.0	(mq)	18	30%
22.0	101.0	599	(mq)	23.0	(mq)	25	30%
8.0	60.0	70	(mq)	<1.0	(mq)	0	0%
8.0	60.0	170	(mq)	11.0	(mq)	0	27%

Food Name	Serving Size	Total Calories
w/sour cream topping	1 serving	400
w/3 oz cheese and bacon	1 serving	780
w/3 oz cheese and broccoli	1 serving	760
POTATO SALAD	1 cup	260
PUDDING		
butterscotch	3.5 oz	140
chocolate	3.5 oz	140
vanilla	3.5 oz	140
RADISH	.5 oz	2
REFRIED BEANS	3 oz	120
RICE, Spanish	3.5 oz	90
ROAST BEEF, 2.8-oz	1 serving	140
ROAST BEEF SANDWICH		
large, 8 oz	1 serving	570
regular, 5.25 oz	1 serving	320
small, 'Uncle Al' 3.1 oz	1 serving	260
SALAD		
chef's, w/o dressing, 12.5 oz	1 serving	230
garden w/o dressing, 10.5 oz	1 serving	160
garden, gourmet 'Lighterside'	1 serving	134
macaroni	3.5 oz	160
pasta	3.5 oz	80
potato	1 cup	260
three-bean	1/2 cup	100
SALAD DRESSING		
blue cheese	1 tbsp	50
blue cheese, 'Lite'	1 tbsp	35
French	1 tbsp	60
Italian	1 tbsp	50
Italian, 'Lite'	1 tbsp	30
oil	1 tbsp	130
poppy seed	1 tbsp	60
ranch	1 tbsp	45

Prot. MGS	Carbs. GMS	Sodium MGS	Fiber GMS	Fat GMS	Sat. Fat GMS	Chol. MGS	% Fat Cal.
11.0	65.0	149	na	11.0	na	tr	25%
22.0	110.0	910	(mq)	28.0	(mq)	23	32%
19.0	112.0	489	(mq)	26.0	(mq)	11	31%
7.0	41.0	127	(mq)	17.0	(mq)	7	59%
2.0	20.0	150	(tr)	6.0	(mq)	2	39%
2.0	20.0	120	(tr)	6.0	(mq)	2	39%
2.0	20.0	120	(tr)	6.0	(mq)	2	39%
<1.0	<1.0	<1	(mq)	<1.0	(tr)	0	0%
6.0	16.0	375	(mq)	4.0	(mq)	2	30%
3.0	20.0	442	(mq)	<1.0	na	0	0%
14.0	<1.0	524	0	9.0	(mq)	36	58%
22.0	41.0	1169	(mq)	35.0	(mq)	36	55%
20.0	33.0	969	(mq)	11.0	(mq)	36	31%
12.0	21.0	562	(mq)	14.0	(mq)	19	48%
22.0	4.0	1048	(mq)	14.0	(mq)	322	55%
12.0	4.0	362	(mq)	11.0	(mq)	273	62%
7.0	13.0	350	na	6.0	na	2	40%
2.0	21.0	216	(mq)	7.0	(mq)	<1	39%
2.0	16.0	322	(mq)	1.0	(mq)	<1	11%
7.0	41.0	tr	(mq)	7.0	(mq)	7	24%
3.0	23.0	450	(mq)	<1.0	(mq)	0	0%
<1.0	1.0	110	na	5.0	(mq)	8	90%
<1.0	2.0	240	na	3.0	(mq)	3	77%
<1.0	6.0	140	na	4.0	(mq)	0	60%
<1.0	3.0	159	na	4.0	(mq)	0	72%
<1.0	1.0	152	na	3.0	(mq)	0	90%
<1.0	<1.0	<1	0	14.0	(mq)	0	97%
<1.0	5.0	107	na	4.0	(mq)	6	60%
<1.0	<1.0	103	na	5.0	(mq)	5	100%

Food Name	Serving Size	Total Calories
Thousand Island	1 tbsp	70
Thousand Island, 'Lite'	1 tbsp	40
vinegar	1 tbsp	2
SOUR CREAM, imitation	3.5 oz	130
SOY NUTS	1 oz	120
SPAGHETTI	3.5 oz	140
SPAGHETTI SAUCE		
regular	3.5 oz	80
w/meat	3.5 oz	150
SPICY MEAT SAUCE	3.5 oz	80
STRAWBERRIES	2 oz	18
SUNFLOWER SEEDS, w/raisins	1 oz	130
TACO SAUCE	3.5 oz	30
TACO SHELL	1 shell	40
TOMATO	1 oz	6
TORTILLA	1 tortilla	110
TORTILLA CHIPS	1 oz	140
TURKEY BITS	2 oz	70
TURKEY SANDWICH, turkey bacon club, 9 oz	1 sandwich	670
WATERMELON	2 pieces	18
WHIPPED TOPPING	1 dollop	50

RED LOBSTER

Food Name	Serving Size	Total Calories
CALAMARI		
breaded, fried, dinner portion, 10 oz	1 serving	720
breaded, fried, 5 oz	1 serving	360
CATFISH		
breast, 4 oz	1 serving	120
dinner portion, 10 oz raw wt	1 serving	340
lunch portion, 5 oz raw wt	1 serving	170

Prot. MGS	Carbs. GMS	Sodium MGS	Fiber GMS	Fat GMS	Sat. Fat GMS	Chol. MGS	% Fat Cal.
<1.0	6.0	110	na	6.0	(mq)	8	77%
<1.0	3.0	143	na	3.0	(mq)	5	68%
<1.0	<1.0	5	0	<1.0	(tr)	0	0%
3.0	5.0	79	na	11.0	(mq)	<1	76%
10.0	5.0	151	(mq)	7.0	(mq)	0	53%
3.0	23.0	1	(mq)	4.0	(mq)	0	26%
1.0	19.0	635	(mq)	<1.0	(mq)	<1	0%
7.0	12.0	419	(mq)	8.0	(mq)	<1	48%
5.0	6.0	751	na	4.0	(mq)	12	45%
<1.0	4.0	<1	(mq)	<1.0	(tr)	0	0%
5.0	6.0	5	(mq)	10.0	(mq)	0	69%
1.0	6.0	806	na	<1.0	(tr)	0	0%
<1.0	6.0	53	(mq)	2.0	(mq)	0	45%
<1.0	2.0	6	(mq)	<1.0	(tr)	0	0%
3.0	19.0	284	(mq)	2.0	(mq)	0	16%
2.0	17.0	100	(mq)	7.0	(mq)	0	45%
10.0	<1.0	686	0	3.0	(mq)	49	39%
29.0	41.0	1878	(mq)	43.0	(mq)	87	58%
<1.0	4.0	<1	(mq)	<1.0	(tr)	0	0%
<1.0	4.0	6	0	4.0	(mq)	2	72%
26.0	60.0	2300	na	42.0	12.0	280	53%
13.0	30.0	1150	na	21.0	6.0	140	53%
24.0	0.0	60	na	3.0	1.0	65	23%
40.0	0.0	100	na	20.0	6.0	170	53%
20.0	0.0	50	na	10.0	3.0	85	53%

Food Name	Serving Size	Total Calories
CLAM		
cherrystone, dinner portion, 10 oz raw wt	1 serving	260
cherrystone, lunch portion, 5 oz raw wt	1 serving	130
COD FILLET		
Atlantic, dinner portion, 10 oz raw wt	1 serving	200
Atlantic, lunch portion, 5 oz raw wt	1 serving	100
CRAB LEGS		
'King' 1 lb	1 serving	170
'Snow' 1 lb	1 serving	150
FLOUNDER		
dinner portion, 10 oz raw wt	1 serving	200
lunch portion, 5 oz raw wt	1 serving	100
GROUPER		
dinner portion, 10 oz raw wt	1 serving	220
lunch portion, 5 oz raw wt	1 serving	110
HADDOCK		
dinner portion, 10 oz raw wt	1 serving	220
lunch portion, 5 oz raw wt	1 serving	110
HALIBUT		
dinner portion, 10 oz raw wt	1 serving	220
lunch portion, 5 oz raw wt	1 serving	110
HAMBURGER, 1/3 lb	1 serving	320
LANGOSTINO		
dinner portion, 10 oz raw wt	1 serving	240
lunch portion, 5 oz raw wt	1 serving	120
LOBSTER		
Maine, 1 1/4 lb	1 serving	240
rock, 1 tail	1 serving	230
MACKEREL		
dinner portion, 10 oz raw wt	1 serving	380
lunch portion, 5 oz raw wt	1 serving	190

Prot. MGS	Carbs. GMS	Sodium MGS	Fiber GMS	Fat GMS	Sat. Fat GMS	Chol. MGS	% Fat Cal.
36.0	22.0	1080	na	4.0	tr	160	14%
18.0	11.0	540	na	2.0	tr	80	14%
46.0	0.0	400	na	2.0	tr	140	9%
23.0	0.0	200	na	1.0	tr	70	9%
32.0	6.0	900	na	2.0	tr	100	11%
33.0	1.0	1630	na	2.0	1.0	130	12%
42.0	2.0	190	na	2.0	tr	140	9%
21.0	1.0	95	na	1.0	tr	70	9%
52.0	0.0	140	na	2.0	tr	130	8%
26.0	0.0	70	na	1.0	tr	65	8%
48.0	4.0	360	na	2.0	tr	170	8%
24.0	2.0	180	na	1.0	tr	85	8%
50.0	2.0	210	na	2.0	tr	120	8%
25.0	1.0	105	na	1.0	tr	60	8%
27.0	0.0	70	na	23.0	11.0	105	65%
52.0	4.0	820	na	2.0	tr	420	8%
26.0	2.0	410	na	1.0	tr	210	8%
36.0	5.0	550	na	8.0	2.0	310	30%
49.0	2.0	1090	na	3.0	1.0	200	12%
2.0	40.0	500	na	24.0	8.0	200	57%
1.0	20.0	250	na	12.0	4.0	100	57%

Food Name	Serving Size	Total Calories
MONKFISH		
dinner portion, 10 oz	1 serving	220
lunch portion, 5 oz	1 serving	110
MUSSEL, 3 oz	1 serving	70
OCEAN PERCH		
Atlantic, dinner portion, 10 oz raw wt ..	1 serving	260
Atlantic, lunch portion, 5 oz raw wt	1 serving	130
OYSTER, raw, on half shell, 6 pieces ...	1 serving	110
POLLACK		
dinner portion, 10 oz raw wt	1 serving	240
lunch portion, 5 oz raw wt	1 serving	120
RED ROCKFISH		
dinner portion, 10 oz raw wt	1 serving	180
lunch portion, 5 oz raw wt	1 serving	90
RED SNAPPER		
dinner portion, 10 oz raw wt	1 serving	220
lunch portion, 5 oz raw wt	1 serving	110
SALMON		
Norwegian, dinner portion, 10 oz raw wt	1 serving	460
Norwegian, lunch portion, 5 oz raw wt	1 serving	230
Sockeye, dinner portion, 10 oz raw wt	1 serving	320
Sockeye, lunch portion, 5 oz raw wt ..	1 serving	160
SCALLOP		
calico, dinner portion, 10 oz raw wt ...	1 serving	360
calico, lunch portion, 5 oz raw wt	1 serving	180
deep sea, dinner portion, 10 oz raw wt	1 serving	260
deep sea, lunch portion, 5 oz raw wt ..	1 serving	130
SHARK		
blacktip, dinner portion, 10 oz raw wt ..	1 serving	300
blacktip, lunch portion, 5 oz raw wt ...	1 serving	150
mako, dinner portion, 10 oz raw wt ...	1 serving	280
mako, lunch portion, 5 oz raw wt	1 serving	140
SHRIMP, 8-12 pieces	1 serving	120

Prot. MGS	Carbs. GMS	Sodium MGS	Fiber GMS	Fat GMS	Sat. Fat GMS	Chol. MGS	% Fat Cal.
0.0	48.0	190	na	2.0	tr	160	8%
0.0	24.0	95	na	1.0	tr	80	8%
9.0	3.0	150	na	2.0	tr	50	26%
48.0	2.0	380	na	8.0	2.0	150	28%
24.0	1.0	190	na	4.0	1.0	75	28%
8.0	11.0	90	na	4.0	2.0	60	33%
56.0	2.0	180	na	2.0	tr	180	8%
28.0	1.0	90	na	1.0	tr	90	8%
42.0	0.0	190	na	2.0	tr	170	10%
21.0	0.0	95	na	1.0	tr	85	10%
50.0	0.0	280	na	2.0	tr	140	8%
25.0	0.0	140	na	1.0	tr	70	8%
54.0	6.0	120	na	24.0	6.0	160	47%
27.0	3.0	60	na	12.0	3.0	80	47%
56.0	6.0	120	na	8.0	2.0	100	23%
28.0	3.0	60	na	4.0	1.0	50	23%
64.0	16.0	320	na	4.0	tr	230	10%
32.0	8.0	260	na	2.0	tr	115	10%
52.0	4.0	520	na	4.0	tr	100	14%
26.0	2.0	260	na	2.0	tr	50	14%
70.0	0.0	180	na	2.0	tr	120	6%
35.0	0.0	90	na	1.0	tr	60	6%
68.0	0.0	120	na	2.0	tr	200	6%
34.0	0.0	60	na	1.0	tr	100	6%
25.0	0.0	110	na	2.0	tr	230	15%

Food Name	Serving Size	Total Calories
SOLE		
lemon, dinner portion, 10 oz raw wt	1 serving	240
lemon, lunch portion, 5 oz raw wt	1 serving	120
STRIP STEAK, 7 oz	1 serving	690
SWORDFISH		
dinner portion, 10 oz raw weight	1 serving	200
lunch portion, 5 oz raw weight	1 serving	100
TILEFISH		
dinner portion, 10 oz raw wt	1 serving	200
lunch portion, 5 oz raw wt	1 serving	100
TROUT		
rainbow, dinner portion, 10 oz raw wt	1 serving	340
rainbow, lunch portion, 5 oz raw wt	1 serving	170
TUNA		
yellowfin, dinner portion, 10 oz raw wt	1 serving	360
yellowfin, lunch portion, 5 oz raw wt	1 serving	180

ROUND TABLE PIZZA

pizza, cheese, pan, large pie	1 slice	310
pizza, cheese, thin crust, large pie	1 slice	166

ROY ROGERS

ALFALFA SPROUTS	2 tbsp	1
BACON BITS	1 tsp	33
BEAN SPROUTS	2 tbsp	4
BEETS, sliced	1/4 cup	18
BISCUIT	1 serving	231
BREAKFAST		
egg and biscuit platter	1 serving	557
egg and biscuit platter, w/bacon	1 serving	607
egg and biscuit platter, w/ham	1 serving	605

Prot. MGS	Carbs. GMS	Sodium MGS	Fiber GMS	Fat GMS	Sat. Fat GMS	Chol. MGS	% Fat Cal.
54.0	2.0	180	na	2.0	tr	130	8%
27.0	1.0	90	na	1.0	tr	65	8%
29.0	0.0	70	na	64.0	27.0	140	83%
34.0	0.0	280	na	8.0	2.0	200	36%
17.0	0.0	140	na	4.0	1.0	100	36%
40.0	0.0	120	na	4.0	2.0	160	18%
20.0	0.0	60	na	2.0	1.0	80	18%
46.0	0.0	180	na	18.0	6.0	180	48%
23.0	0.0	90	na	9.0	3.0	90	48%
64.0	0.0	140	na	12.0	4.0	140	30%
32.0	0.0	70	na	6.0	2.0	70	30%
13.0	40.0	631	na	11.0	na	30	32%
8.0	18.0	332	na	7.0	na	21	38%
tr	tr	<1	(mq)	tr	(tr)	0	0%
3.0	2.0	189	na	1.0	na	0	27%
tr	1.0	<1	(mq)	tr	(tr)	0	0%
1.0	4.0	162	(mq)	tr	(tr)	0	0%
4.0	26.0	575	(mq)	12.0	(mq)	5	47%
18.0	44.0	1020	(mq)	34.0	(mq)	417	55%
21.0	44.0	1236	(mq)	39.0	(mq)	424	58%
25.0	44.0	1442	(mq)	36.0	(mq)	437	54%

Food Name	Serving Size	Total Calories
egg and biscuit platter, w/sausage	1 serving	713
pancake platter, w/syrup and butter ...	1 serving	386
pancake platter, w/syrup and butter, w/bacon	1 serving	436
pancake platter, w/syrup and butter, w/ham	1 serving	434
pancake platter, w/syrup and butter, w/sausage	1 serving	542
BREAKFAST SANDWICH		
crescent	1 serving	408
crescent, w/bacon	1 serving	446
crescent, w/ham	1 serving	456
crescent, w/sausage	1 serving	564
BROCCOLI, raw	1/4 cup	6
CABBAGE, raw	1/4 cup	5
CANTALOUPE, cubed	1/4 cup	14
CARROT, raw, shredded	1/4 cup	12
CAULIFLOWER, raw	1/4 cup	6
CHEESE, cheddar	1/4 cup	100
CHEESEBURGER		
'Express'	1 serving	613
'Express' w/bacon	1 serving	641
regular	1 serving	525
small	1 serving	275
w/bacon	1 serving	552
CHICKEN		
breast, fried	1 serving	412
breast and wing, fried	1 serving	604
breast and wing, w/o skin, 'Roy's Roaster'	1 serving	190
leg, fried	1 serving	140
leg and thigh, fried	1 serving	436
nugget, fried, 6 pieces	1 serving	288

Prot. MGS	Carbs. GMS	Sodium MGS	Fiber GMS	Fat GMS	Sat. Fat GMS	Chol. MGS	% Fat Cal.
25.0	44.0	1345	(mq)	49.0	(mq)	458	62%
5.0	63.0	547	(mq)	13.0	(mq)	51	30%
8.0	63.0	763	(mq)	17.0	(mq)	58	35%
11.0	64.0	969	(mq)	15.0	(mq)	71	31%
11.0	63.0	872	(mq)	28.0	(mq)	92	46%
13.0	28.0	820	(mq)	27.0	(mq)	207	60%
15.0	28.0	982	(mq)	30.0	(mq)	212	61%
20.0	29.0	1243	(mq)	29.0	(mq)	227	57%
19.0	28.0	1145	(mq)	42.0	(mq)	248	67%
1.0	1.0	6	(mq)	tr	(tr)	0	0%
tr	1.0	2	(mq)	tr	(tr)	0	0%
tr	3.0	4	(mq)	tr	(tr)	0	0%
tr	3.0	2	(mq)	tr	(tr)	0	0%
1.0	1.0	4	(mq)	tr	(tr)	0	0%
7.0	tr	275	0	8.0	(mq)	15	72%
30.0	42.0	1122	(mq)	37.0	(mq)	82	54%
33.0	36.0	1317	(mq)	41.0	(mq)	89	58%
29.0	37.0	830	(mq)	29.0	(mq)	76	50%
15.0	24.0	558	(mq)	13.0	(mq)	36	43%
32.0	31.0	1025	(mq)	33.0	(mq)	83	54%
33.0	17.0	609	(mq)	24.0	(mq)	118	52%
44.0	25.0	894	(mq)	37.0	(mq)	165	55%
32.0	2.0	na	na	6.0	na	na	28%
12.0	6.0	190	(mq)	8.0	(mq)	40	51%
30.0	17.0	596	(mq)	28.0	(mq)	125	58%
10.0	21.0	548	(mq)	18.0	(mq)	63	56%

Food Name	Serving Size	Total Calories
thigh, fried	1 serving	296
wing, fried	1 serving	192
CHICKEN SALAD, grilled	1 serving	120
CHINESE NOODLES	1/4 cup	55
COLESLAW	1 serving	110
COTTAGE CHEESE	2 tbsp	29
CROUTONS	2 tbsp	14
CUCUMBER, raw	5-6 slices	4
DANISH		
apple swirl	1 serving	328
cheese swirl	1 serving	383
EGG, boiled, chopped	2 tbsp	55
FISH SANDWICH	1 serving	514
FRENCH FRIES		
large order, 5.5 oz	1 serving	440
regular order, 4 oz	1 serving	320
small order, 3 oz	1 serving	238
FRUIT COCKTAIL	1/4 cup	46
GARBANZO BEANS	1/4 cup	55
GELATIN, parfait	1/4 cup	50
GRANOLA	1/4 cup	65
GRAPES	5 grapes	20
GREEK PASTA	1/4 cup	159
HAMBURGER		
'Express'	1 serving	561
regular	1 serving	472
'Roy Rogers Bar'	1 serving	573
small	1 serving	222
HONEYDEW MELON, cubed	1/4 cup	15
LEMONADE	12 oz	150
LETTUCE		
iceberg	1 cup	7
romaine	1 cup	9

Prot. MGS	Carbs. GMS	Sodium MGS	Fiber GMS	Fat GMS	Sat. Fat GMS	Chol. MGS	% Fat Cal.
18.0	12.0	406	(mq)	20.0	(mq)	85	61%
11.0	9.0	285	(mq)	13.0	(mq)	47	61%
18.0	2.0	520	na	4.0	na	60	30%
2.0	7.0	113	(mq)	3.0	(mq)	1	49%
1.0	11.0	261	(mq)	7.0	(mq)	5	57%
4.0	<1.0	114	0	1.0	(mq)	4	31%
1.0	3.0	50	(mq)	tr	(tr)	0	0%
tr	1.0	2	(mq)	0.0	0.0	0	0%
5.0	62.0	279	(mq)	7.0	(mq)	na	19%
8.0	54.0	369	(mq)	15.0	(mq)	na	35%
4.0	1.0	41	0	4.0	(mq)	(mq)	65%
18.0	58.0	857	(mq)	24.0	(mq)	62	42%
6.0	54.0	225	(mq)	22.0	(mq)	19	45%
4.0	39.0	164	(mq)	16.0	(mq)	13	45%
3.0	29.0	122	(mq)	12.0	(mq)	10	45%
tr	12.0	1	(mq)	tr	(tr)	0	0%
3.0	9.0	240	(mq)	1.0	(mq)	0	16%
1.0	10.0	23	(tr)	2.0	(mq)	0	36%
2.0	9.0	8	(mq)	3.0	(mq)	0	42%
tr	5.0	<1	(mq)	tr	(tr)	0	0%
3.0	19.0	328	(mq)	9.0	(mq)	na	51%
27.0	42.0	899	(mq)	32.0	(mq)	70	51%
26.0	37.0	607	(mq)	25.0	(mq)	64	48%
36.0	38.0	1252	(mq)	31.0	(mq)	96	49%
12.0	23.0	336	(mq)	9.0	(mq)	26	36%
tr	4.0	4	(mq)	tr	(tr)	0	0%
tr	39.0	na	na	tr	na	na	0%
1.0	1.0	5	(mq)	tr	(tr)	0	0%
1.0	1.0	5	(mq)	tr	(tr)	0	0%

Food Name	Serving Size	Total Calories
MACARONI SALAD	1/4 cup	93
MILK, 2%	8 oz	120
MILKSHAKE		
chocolate	1 serving	358
strawberry	1 serving	315
vanilla	1 serving	306
ONION, raw, chopped	2 tbsp	7
ORANGE JUICE	8 oz	120
PASTA AND NOODLES. See individual listings.		
PASTRY, cinnamon rod	1 serving	376
PEACH, sliced	1/4 cup	48
PEAS, green	1/4 cup	28
PEPPER, GREEN	2 tbsp	3
PINEAPPLE		
chunks, canned	1/4 cup	48
chunks, fresh	1/4 cup	19
POTATO, BAKED, plain 'Hot Topped'	1 serving	211
POTATO SALAD	1/4 cup	54
RADISH, sliced	2 tbsp	2
ROAST BEEF SANDWICH		
large	1 serving	373
large, w/cheese	1 serving	427
regular	1 serving	350
w/cheese	1 serving	403
ROLL, crescent	1 serving	287
SALAD DRESSING		
bacon and tomato	2 tbsp	136
blue cheese	2 tbsp	150
Italian, low-calorie	2 tbsp	70
ranch	2 tbsp	155
Thousand Island	2 tbsp	160
STRAWBERRIES, fresh	1/4 cup	11

Prot. MGS	Carbs. GMS	Sodium MGS	Fiber GMS	Fat GMS	Sat. Fat GMS	Chol. MGS	% Fat Cal.
2.0	10.0	301	(mq)	5.0	(mq)	na	48%
8.0	11.0	130	na	5.0	na	18	38%
8.0	61.0	290	(tr)	10.0	(mq)	37	25%
8.0	49.0	261	(tr)	10.0	(mq)	37	29%
8.0	45.0	282	0	11.0	(mq)	40	32%
tr	2.0	tr	(mq)	tr	(tr)	0	0%
2.0	32.0	na	na	tr	na	na	0%
5.0	55.0	339	(mq)	15.0	(mq)	na	36%
tr	13.0	5	(mq)	tr	(tr)	0	0%
2.0	5.0	41	(mq)	tr	(tr)	0	0%
tr	1.0	tr	(mq)	tr	(tr)	0	0%
tr	12.0	5	(mq)	tr	(tr)	0	0%
tr	5.0	<1	(mq)	tr	(tr)	0	0%
6.0	48.0	65	na	0.0	na	0	0%
1.0	5.0	348	(mq)	3.0	(mq)	na	50%
tr	1.0	4	(mq)	tr	(tr)	0	0%
35.0	31.0	840	(mq)	12.0	(mq)	82	29%
38.0	31.0	1062	(mq)	17.0	(mq)	94	36%
26.0	37.0	732	(mq)	11.0	(mq)	68	28%
29.0	37.0	954	(mq)	15.0	(mq)	70	33%
5.0	27.0	547	(mq)	18.0	(mq)	5	56%
tr	6.0	150	na	12.0	(mq)	na	79%
2.0	2.0	153	na	16.0	(mq)	na	96%
0.0	2.0	100	na	6.0	na	na	77%
tr	4.0	100	na	14.0	(mq)	na	81%
tr	4.0	150	na	16.0	(mq)	na	90%
tr	3.0	<1	(mq)	tr	(tr)	0	0%

Food Name	Serving Size	Total Calories
SUNDAE		
caramel	1 serving	293
chocolate	1 serving	358
hot fudge	1 serving	337
strawberry	1 serving	216
vanilla	1 serving	306
TOMATO	3 slices	20
WATERMELON, diced	1/4 cup	13

SHAKEY'S PIZZA

CHICKEN ENTRÉE		
5 pieces, fried, w/potatoes	1 serving	1700
3 pieces, fried, w/potatoes	1 serving	947
HAM AND CHEESE SANDWICH,		
'Hot Ham & Cheese'	1 sandwich	550
HERO SANDWICH, 'Super Hot Hero'	1 sandwich	810
PIZZA		
cheese, 'Homestyle Pan Crust' 12-inch pie	1/10 pie	303
cheese, thick crust, 12-inch pie	1/10 pie	170
cheese, thin crust, 12-inch pie	1/10 pie	133
pepperoni, 'Homestyle Pan Crust' 12-inch pie	1/10 pie	343
pepperoni, thick crust, 12-inch pie	1/10 pie	185
pepperoni, thin crust, 12-inch pie	1/10 pie	148
sausage and mushroom, 'Homestyle Pan Crust' 12-inch pie	1/10 pie	343
sausage and mushroom, thick crust, 12-inch pie	1/10 pie	179
sausage and mushroom, thin crust, 12-inch pie	1/10 pie	141

Prot. MGS	Carbs. GMS	Sodium MGS	Fiber GMS	Fat GMS	Sat. Fat GMS	Chol. MGS	% Fat Cal.
7.0	52.0	193	(tr)	9.0	(mq)	23	28%
8.0	61.0	290	na	10.0	na	37	25%
7.0	53.0	186	(tr)	13.0	(mq)	23	35%
6.0	33.0	99	(tr)	7.0	(mq)	23	29%
8.0	45.0	282	na	11.0	na	40	32%
1.0	5.0	1	(mq)	tr	(tr)	0	0%
tr	3.0	1	(mq)	tr	(tr)	0	0%
97.0	130.0	5327	(mq)	90.0	(mq)	(mq)	48%
57.0	51.0	2293	(mq)	56.0	(mq)	(mq)	53%
36.0	56.0	2135	na	21.0	na	na	34%
36.0	67.0	2688	(mq)	44.0	(mq)	(mq)	49%
14.1	31.0	591	(mq)	13.7	(mq)	21	41%
9.0	21.6	421	(mq)	4.8	(mq)	13	25%
8.4	13.2	323	(mq)	5.2	(mq)	14	35%
15.8	31.1	740	(mq)	15.4	(mq)	27	40%
10.1	21.8	422	(mq)	6.4	(mq)	17	31%
8.4	13.2	403	(mq)	6.9	(mq)	14	42%
16.4	31.4	677	(mq)	16.9	(mq)	24	44%
10.2	21.8	420	(mq)	5.6	(mq)	15	28%
8.5	13.3	336	(mq)	6.0	(mq)	13	38%

Food Name	Serving Size	Total Calories
sausage and pepperoni, 'Homestyle Pan Crust' 12-inch pie	1/10 pie	374
sausage and pepperoni, thick crust, 12-inch pie	1/10 pie	177
sausage and pepperoni, thin crust, 12-inch pie	1/10 pie	166
'Shakey's Special' 'Homestyle Pan Crust' 12-inch pie	1/10 pie	384
'Shakey's Special' thick crust, 12-inch pie	1/10 pie	208
'Shakey's Special' thin crust, 12-inch pie	1/10 pie	171
vegetable, 'Homestyle Pan Crust' 12-inch pie	1/10 pie	320
vegetable, thick crust, 12-inch pie	1/10 pie	162
vegetable, thin crust, 12-inch pie	1/10 pie	125
POTATO WEDGES	15 pieces	950
SPAGHETTI ENTRÉE, w/meat sauce and garlic bread	1 serving	940

SHONEY'S

Food Name	Serving Size	Total Calories
BARBECUE SAUCE, soufflé cup	1 serving	41
BEAN SOUP	6 oz	63
BEEF SOUP, w/cabbage	6 oz	86
BISCUIT	1 serving	170
BREAD, Grecian	1 serving	80
BREAKFAST		
bacon	3 strips	109
egg, fried	1 egg	159
grits	3 oz	57
ham	2 slices	59
pancake, 6-inch diam	1 pancake	91
sausage	1 patty	103

Prot. MGS	Carbs. GMS	Sodium MGS	Fiber GMS	Fat GMS	Sat. Fat GMS	Chol. MGS	% Fat Cal.
17.4	31.2	676	(mq)	19.9	(mq)	24	48%
11.1	21.7	424	(mq)	8.0	(mq)	19	41%
9.4	13.2	397	(mq)	8.4	(mq)	17	46%
17.9	31.6	878	(mq)	20.7	(mq)	29	49%
13.1	22.3	423	(mq)	8.3	(mq)	18	36%
13.3	13.5	475	(mq)	8.7	(mq)	16	46%
14.7	32.1	652	(mq)	14.7	(mq)	21	41%
9.1	22.2	418	(mq)	4.1	(mq)	13	23%
7.2	13.8	313	(mq)	4.5	(mq)	11	32%
17.0	120.0	3703	(mq)	36.0	(mq)	na	34%
26.0	134.0	1904	(mq)	33.0	(mq)	(mq)	32%
0.1	8.2	232	0	1.0	na	0	22%
3.8	9.8	479	1.4	1.1	(mq)	4	16%
6.1	9.4	503	2.3	3.0	(mq)	13	31%
2.7	21.6	364	0	8.1	(mq)	0	43%
2.0	13.2	94	0	2.2	(mq)	0	25%
5.8	0.1	303	0	9.4	(mq)	16	78%
6.1	0.6	69	0	14.7	(mq)	274	83%
0.7	6.2	62	0	3.2	(mq)	0	51%
7.2	0.6	526	0	2.1	(mq)	28	32%
1.8	19.9	522	0	0.2	(mq)	0	2%
3.7	0.2	161	0	9.6	(mq)	17	84%

Food Name	Serving Size	Total Calories
BROCCOLI SOUP, cream of	6 oz	75
BROCCOLI-CAULIFLOWER SOUP	6 oz	124
BROWNIE, walnut, à la mode	1 serving	576
CAKE		
carrot	1 serving	500
hot fudge	1 serving	522
CHEESE SANDWICH		
grilled	1 sandwich	454
grilled, w/bacon	1 sandwich	440
CHEESE SOUP, Florentine, w/ham	6 oz	110
CHEESEBURGER		
'Mushroom/Swiss Burger'	1 sandwich	616
patty melt	1 sandwich	640
CHICKEN ENTRÉE		
charbroiled, 'LightSide'	1 serving	239
tenders, 'America's Favorites'	1 serving	388
CHICKEN SANDWICH		
charbroiled	1 sandwich	451
fillet	1 sandwich	464
CHICKEN GUMBO	6 oz	60
CHICKEN NOODLE SOUP	6 oz	62
CHICKEN RICE SOUP	6 oz	72
CHICKEN SOUP, cream of	6 oz	136
CHICKEN VEGETABLE SOUP, cream of	6 oz	79
CHOWDER		
cheddar	6 oz	91
clam	6 oz	94
corn	6 oz	148
COCKTAIL SAUCE, soufflé cup	1 serving	36
COMBINATION ENTRÉE		
'Fish N' Shrimp'	1 serving	487
shrimp, charbroiled 'Steak N' Shrimp'	1 serving	361
shrimp, fried 'Steak N' Shrimp'	1 serving	507

Prot. MGS	Carbs. GMS	Sodium MGS	Fiber GMS	Fat GMS	Sat. Fat GMS	Chol. MGS	% Fat Cal.
1.8	10.5	415	.4	4.6	(mq)	1	55%
3.8	11.9	560	.5	9.2	(mq)	12	67%
9.6	60.6	435	0	33.7	(mq)	35	53%
9.0	56.0	476	0	26.0	(mq)	37	47%
7.4	81.9	485	0	19.7	(mq)	27	34%
17.0	29.0	1519	na	29.0	na	na	57%
18.2	27.9	1200	1.3	28.2	(mq)	36	58%
3.7	11.8	890	.6	7.8	(mq)	11	64%
31.6	28.8	1135	.7	41.7	(mq)	106	61%
38.8	29.5	826	6.7	41.7	(mq)	121	59%
39.0	1.0	592	na	7.0	na	85	26%
34.9	16.6	239	0	20.4	(mq)	64	47%
43.2	28.1	1002	.5	17.0	(mq)	90	34%
29.7	38.9	585	.5	21.2	(mq)	51	41%
4.0	7.0	1050	na	2.0	(mq)	(mq)	30%
3.1	9.2	127	na	1.4	(mq)	14	20%
3.0	13.3	117	.5	0.5	(mq)	6	6%
4.6	13.5	1164	.3	8.9	(mq)	11	59%
3.5	13.4	714	na	1.3	(mq)	(mq)	15%
3.0	14.4	948	na	2.3	(mq)	(mq)	23%
1.7	9.6	66	0	5.4	(mq)	0	52%
4.0	22.1	510	0	4.7	(mq)	na	29%
0.4	8.7	260	0	0.1	na	0	3%
28.1	36.5	644	.3	25.5	(mq)	127	47%
36.5	1.0	198	0	22.6	(mq)	141	56%
36.5	15.0	249	.1	32.7	(mq)	150	58%

Food Name	Serving Size	Total Calories
rib eye steak and chicken, charbroiled	1 serving	605
sirloin steak and chicken, charbroiled	1 serving	357
steak, charbroiled, and Hawaiian chicken	1 serving	262
steak and chicken, charbroiled	1 serving	239
steak and chicken, charbroiled, 8 oz	1 serving	435
CROISSANT	1 serving	260
FISH		
baked, 'LightSide'	1 serving	170
fried, 'Light'	1 serving	297
FISH AND CHIPS ENTRÉE, w/fries	1 serving	639
FISH SANDWICH	1 sandwich	323
FRENCH FRIES		
4-oz order	1 serving	252
3-oz order	1 serving	189
home fries, 3 oz	1 serving	115
GRAVY, country	3 oz	114
HAM SANDWICH		
baked	1 sandwich	290
club, on whole wheat	1 sandwich	642
HAMBURGER		
'All-American'	1 sandwich	501
'Old-Fashioned Burger'	1 sandwich	470
'Shoney Burger'	1 sandwich	498
w/bacon	1 sandwich	591
HAMBURGER PATTY, beef, light	1 serving	289
ITALIAN FEAST ENTRÉE	1 serving	500
LASAGNA ENTRÉE		
'America's Favorites'	1 serving	297
'LightSide'	1 serving	297
LIVER AND ONIONS ENTRÉE, 'America's Favorites'	1 serving	411
MUSHROOMS, sautéed	3 oz	75

Prot. MGS	Carbs. GMS	Sodium MGS	Fiber GMS	Fat GMS	Sat. Fat GMS	Chol. MGS	% Fat Cal.
35.2	0.0	211	0	50.5	(mq)	141	75%
31.9	0.0	160	0	24.5	(mq)	99	62%
39.1	7.4	593	.3	7.4	(mq)	85	25%
39.0	1.3	592	0	7.4	(mq)	85	28%
31.1	0.0	280	0	34.4	(mq)	123	71%
5.0	22.0	260	0	16.0	(mq)	2	55%
35.0	2.0	1641	0	1.0	na	83	5%
19.8	21.5	536	.1	14.4	(mq)	65	44%
32.3	50.4	873	2.9	34.8	na	103	49%
12.2	41.0	740	.4	12.7	(mq)	21	35%
3.9	38.6	364	3.6	9.9	(mq)	0	35%
2.9	28.9	273	2.7	7.5	(mq)	0	36%
2.0	18.7	53	0	3.7	(mq)	0	29%
1.2	5.7	358	0	9.8	(mq)	2	77%
19.2	28.2	1263	1.8	10.3	(mq)	42	32%
37.0	45.2	2105	10.5	35.5	(mq)	78	50%
25.0	26.8	597	.5	32.6	(mq)	86	59%
25.1	25.6	681	.6	28.2	(mq)	82	54%
23.4	22.2	782	.2	35.7	(mq)	79	65%
28.7	28.6	801	.5	40.0	(mq)	86	61%
20.7	0.0	187	0	22.9	(mq)	82	71%
37.5	43.8	369	1.1	19.6	(mq)	74	35%
8.3	44.9	870	2.8	9.8	(mq)	26	30%
8.0	45.0	870	na	10.0	na	26	30%
34.9	15.4	321	.8	22.9	(mq)	529	50%
1.6	4.3	968	1.3	6.5	(mq)	0	78%

Food Name	Serving Size	Total Calories
ONION, sautéed	2.5 oz	37
ONION RINGS	1 ring	52
ONION SOUP	6 oz	29
PASTA AND NOODLES. See SALAD and individual listings.		
PASTRY, honey bun	1 bun	265
PIE		
apple, 'À la mode'	1 serving	492
strawberry	1 serving	332
POTATO, BAKED	10 oz	264
POTATO SOUP	6 oz	102
POTATOES, HASH BROWN	3 oz	90
REUBEN SANDWICH	1 sandwich	596
RICE, 3.5 oz	1 serving	137
SALAD		
ambrosia	1/4 cup	75
apple grape surprise	1/4 cup	19
beet onion	1/4 cup	25
broccoli cauliflower	1/4 cup	98
broccoli cauliflower carrot	1/4 cup	53
broccoli cauliflower ranch	1/4 cup	65
carrot apple	1/4 cup	99
coleslaw	1/4 cup	69
cucumber, lite	1/4 cup	12
Don's pasta	1/4 cup	82
fruit delight	1/4 cup	54
Italian vegetable	1/4 cup	11
kidney bean	1/4 cup	55
macaroni	1/4 cup	207
mixed fruit	1/4 cup	37
mixed squash	1/4 cup	49
Oriental	1/4 cup	79
pea	1/4 cup	73
rotelli pasta	1/4 cup	78

Prot. MGS	Carbs. GMS	Sodium MGS	Fiber GMS	Fat GMS	Sat. Fat GMS	Chol. MGS	% Fat Cal.
0.8	4.3	221	.5	2.1	(mq)	0	51%
0.9	5.0	102	.4	3.1	(mq)	2	54%
1.1	1.5	88	.1	2.0	(mq)	1	62%
4.0	32.0	33	0	14.0	(mq)	3	48%
6.0	67.0	574	na	23.0	(mq)	35	42%
2.1	44.5	247	2.3	16.7	(mq)	0	45%
5.6	61.1	16	6.8	0.3	na	0	1%
1.4	16.8	335	1.6	3.4	(mq)	0	30%
1.6	14.1	50	0	3.1	(mq)	0	31%
32.7	31.5	3873	6.3	34.7	(mq)	138	52%
2.4	23.1	765	.1	3.7	(mq)	1	24%
0.8	11.5	167	.8	3.3	(mq)	0	40%
0.0	4.9	2	.1	0.0	0.0	0	0%
0.6	3.0	167	.8	1.3	(mq)	0	47%
2.3	4.0	478	.9	8.5	(mq)	0	78%
1.1	2.7	193	.9	4.4	(mq)	1	75%
0.9	1.6	12	.9	6.4	(mq)	9	89%
0.6	4.2	10	.9	9.1	(mq)	8	83%
1.1	5.1	106	.9	5.1	(mq)	7	67%
0.2	2.7	344	.2	0.1	na	0	8%
1.8	8.6	223	.2	4.6	(mq)	0	50%
0.6	10.1	2	.7	1.6	(mq)	0	27%
0.4	2.5	110	.7	0.1	na	0	8%
2.6	6.8	154	1.9	2.1	(mq)	2	34%
4.2	17.0	382	.2	13.9	(mq)	14	60%
0.4	9.3	3	.2	0.1	na	0	2%
1.1	2.3	230	.3	4.1	(mq)	0	75%
0.8	13.4	31	.5	2.7	(mq)	1	31%
2.5	3.5	89	2.4	5.5	(mq)	42	68%
1.4	8.9	82	.2	4.0	(mq)	0	46%

Food Name	Serving Size	Total Calories
Seigan	1/4 cup	72
snow	1/4 cup	72
spaghetti	1/4 cup	81
spring	1/4 cup	38
summer	1/4 cup	114
three bean	1/4 cup	96
Waldorf	1/4 cup	81
SALAD DRESSING		
Biscayne, low-calorie	2 tbsp	62
blue cheese	2 tbsp	113
French	2 tbsp	124
French, rue	2 tbsp	122
honey mustard	2 tbsp	165
Italian, creamy	2 tbsp	135
Italian, golden	2 tbsp	141
Italian, nonfat	2 tbsp	10
ranch	2 tbsp	95
Thousand Island	2 tbsp	130
SEAFOOD ENTRÉE, platter	1 serving	566
SHRIMP		
bite-size	1 serving	387
charbroiled	1 serving	138
SHRIMP ENTRÉE		
boiled	1 serving	93
sampler	1 serving	412
'Shrimper's Feast'	1 serving	383
'Shrimper's Feast' large	1 serving	575
SIRLOIN STEAK, charbroiled	6 oz	357
SLIM JIM SANDWICH	1 sandwich	484
SPAGHETTI ENTRÉE		
'America's Favorites'	1 serving	496
'LightSide'	1 serving	248

Prot. MGS	Carbs. GMS	Sodium MGS	Fiber GMS	Fat GMS	Sat. Fat GMS	Chol. MGS	% Fat Cal.
2.3	8.1	122	1.2	3.6	(mq)	5	45%
0.6	9.0	18	.1	4.1	(mq)	0	51%
1.6	8.7	20	.2	4.6	(mq)	0	51%
0.8	2.4	162	.7	2.9	(mq)	0	69%
1.1	2.2	233	.9	11.6	(mq)	0	92%
1.4	11.9	189	1.3	5.1	(mq)	0	48%
0.9	8.5	68	.8	5.2	(mq)	2	58%
6.0	1.0	334	0	1.0	na	0	15%
0.0	0.0	109	0	12.6	(mq)	15	100%
2.0	2.0	204	0	12.0	(mq)	12	87%
5.0	2.0	364	0	10.0	(mq)	0	74%
2.4	2.4	5	0	17.0	(mq)	18	93%
0.0	1.0	454	0	14.5	(mq)	0	97%
0.0	1.0	302	0	15.0	(mq)	0	96%
0.0	2.4	615	0	0.0	0.0	0	0%
0.0	0.0	10	0	10.0	(mq)	15	95%
1.0	2.0	179	0	13.0	(mq)	12	90%
32.8	45.7	893	.3	28.0	(mq)	127	45%
16.4	24.7	1266	0	24.7	(mq)	140	57%
24.7	3.0	170	0	3.0	(mq)	162	20%
19.6	0.0	210	0	1.0	(mq)	182	10%
25.5	26.1	783	.1	22.7	(mq)	217	50%
16.5	29.9	216	.3	22.2	(mq)	125	52%
24.8	44.9	324	.4	33.3	(mq)	188	52%
31.9	0.0	160	0	24.5	(mq)	99	62%
27.4	40.4	1620	.5	23.9	(mq)	57	44%
24.2	63.4	387	2.2	16.3	(mq)	55	30%
12.0	32.0	194	na	8.0	na	28	29%

Food Name	Serving Size	Total Calories
STEAK ENTRÉE, country-fried, 'America's Favorites'	1 serving	449
STEAK SANDWICH		
country-fried	1 sandwich	588
Philly	1 sandwich	673
SUNDAE		
hot fudge	1 serving	451
strawberry	1 serving	380
SWEET AND SOUR SAUCE, soufflé cup	1 serving	58
SYRUP, low-calorie	2.2 oz	98
TARTAR SAUCE, soufflé cup	1 serving	84
TOAST, buttered	2 slices	163
TOMATO SOUP		
Florentine	6 oz	63
vegetable	6 oz	46
TURKEY SANDWICH, turkey club, on whole wheat	1 sandwich	635
VEGETABLE BEEF SOUP	6 oz	82

SIZZLER

Food Name	Serving Size	Total Calories
ALFALFA SPROUTS	1/4 cup	2
AVOCADO	1/2 avocado	153
BACON BITS	1 tbsp	27
BEAN SPROUTS	1/4 cup	8
BEANS		
garbanzo	1/4 cup	63
kidney	1/4 cup	52
BEEF PATTY		
ground, 8-oz size	1 serving	530
ground, 5.33-oz size	1 serving	353
BEETS	1/4 cup	13
BREAD, focaccia	2 pieces	108

Prot. MGS	Carbs. GMS	Sodium MGS	Fiber GMS	Fat GMS	Sat. Fat GMS	Chol. MGS	% Fat Cal.
19.4	33.9	1177	.9	27.2	(mq)	27	55%
24.5	67.0	1501	1.4	25.8	(mq)	29	39%
31.8	37.2	1242	.1	44.0	(mq)	103	59%
7.0	60.0	226	0	22.0	(mq)	60	44%
6.0	47.7	145	.3	19.0	(mq)	69	45%
0.0	14.7	5	0	0.0	0.0	0	0%
0.0	24.4	0	0	0.0	0.0	0	0%
0.2	3.6	177	0	7.7	(mq)	11	83%
4.2	24.6	296	1.2	5.2	(mq)	0	29%
2.3	11.0	683	0	1.1	(mq)	0	16%
1.9	9.8	314	.4	0.3	(mq)	0	6%
43.5	44.1	1289	10.2	32.7	(mq)	100	46%
3.5	14.1	1254	.3	1.5	(mq)	5	16%
0.0	0.0	0	0	0.0	0.0	0	0%
2.0	6.0	11	3.0	15.0	2.0	0	88%
2.0	2.0	165	1.0	2.0	0.0	0	67%
1.0	2.0	2	0	0.0	0.0	0	0%
3.0	11.0	255	3.0	1.0	0.0	0	14%
3.0	10.0	222	4.0	0.0	0.0	0	0%
42.0	0.0	150	na	38.0	15.4	156	65%
28.0	0.0	100	na	28.0	10.2	104	71%
0.0	3.0	117	1.0	0.0	0.0	0	0%
2.0	9.0	134	0	7.0	1.0	1	58%

Food Name	Serving Size	Total Calories
BREADSTICKS, garlic, soft	1 oz	75
BROCCOLI, raw	1/2 cup	12
BROCCOLI CHEESE SOUP	4 oz	139
CABBAGE, red, raw	1/4 cup	5
CANTALOUPE	1/2 cup	28
CARROTS, raw	1/4 cup	12
CAULIFLOWER, battered, unprepared, approx 3.5 oz	1 serving	184
CHEESE		
cheddar, imitation, shredded	1 oz	85
Parmesan, grated	1 oz	110
Swiss, sliced	1 oz	100
CHEESE SAUCE, nacho	2 oz	120
CHEESE TOAST	1 slice	273
CHICKEN		
breast, lemon herb	5 oz	151
patty, Malibu	1 patty	368
wings	1 oz	73
wings, disjointed, Cajun	3 oz	201
wings, disjointed, Southern style	1 oz	73
wings, whole, Southern style	1 oz	74
CHICKEN ENTRÉE, w/noodles	6 oz	164
CHICKEN NOODLE SOUP	4 oz	31
CHICKEN STRIPS, breaded	1 oz	68
CHILI, w/beans, 'Grande'	6 oz	100
CHOCOLATE SYRUP	1 oz	90
CHOWDER, clam	4 oz	118
COCKTAIL SAUCE	1.5 oz	40
CORN NUGGETS	3 oz	117
CORNED BEEF, sliced	1 oz	45
COTTAGE CHEESE		
low-fat	1/2 cup	100
regular	2 oz	51

Prot. MGS	Carbs. GMS	Sodium MGS	Fiber GMS	Fat GMS	Sat. Fat GMS	Chol. MGS	% Fat Cal.
2.3	15.2	112	na	0.5	na	na	6%
1.0	2.0	12	1.0	0.0	0.0	0	0%
3.0	10.0	355	0	9.0	2.0	8	58%
0.0	1.0	2	0	0.0	0.0	0	0%
1.0	7.0	7	1.0	0.0	0.0	0	0%
0.0	3.0	10	1.0	0.0	0.0	0	0%
3.1	21.1	49	na	10.3	0.0	1	50%
2.0	4.5	375	na	6.5	1.5	0	69%
11.0	2.0	550	na	7.0	4.8	4	57%
8.0	1.0	74	na	8.0	na	25	72%
5.0	3.0	600	0	10.0	5.0	30	75%
6.0	16.0	494	1.0	21.0	5.0	5	69%
27.0	27.0	na	na	4.0	na	na	24%
27.0	12.0	na	na	25.0	na	na	61%
4.0	4.0	136	0	4.0	1.0	20	49%
15.9	1.8	435	na	14.4	na	111	64%
4.7	3.7	135	na	6.0	1.1	20	74%
3.9	3.7	285	na	4.8	1.7	18	58%
13.0	20.0	524	na	4.0	0.7	40	22%
2.0	4.0	495	0	1.0	0.0	7	29%
3.6	na	130	na	4.6	0.9	9	61%
5.0	18.0	1190	na	1.0	na	0	9%
0.0	21.0	15	0	0.0	0.0	0	0%
3.0	11.0	511	0	6.0	0.0	6	46%
0.0	8.0	396	0	0.0	0.0	0	0%
2.5	22.0	325	na	8.4	na	0	65%
7.5	0.2	55	na	1.5	na	na	30%
14.0	4.0	390	na	2.0	1.0	8	18%
8.0	2.0	230	0	1.0	1.0	5	18%

Food Name	Serving Size	Total Calories
CRAB		
imitation, shredded, approx 3.5 oz	1 serving	104
snow, legs and claws, scored	3.5 oz	91
CRACKER, saltine	2 crackers	25
CREAMER, nondairy	.5 oz	12
CROISSANT, mini	1 croissant	120
CUCUMBER, raw	2 oz	7
DESSERT, parfait salad, approx 3.5 oz	1 serving	84
EGG		
cooked, diced	2 oz	85
cooked, salad topping	1 oz	44
FETTUCCINE, whole egg	2 oz	80
FILET MIGNON STEAK, 7 oz	3 oz	179
FISH NUGGETS	1 oz	40
FRENCH FRIES	4 oz	358
GRAPES	1/2 cup	29
GUACAMOLE		
extra chunky, approx 3.5 oz	1 serving	285
regular	1 oz	42
HALIBUT STEAK		
8-oz size	1 serving	240
6-oz size	1 serving	180
HAMBURGER, w/lettuce and tomato	1 serving	626
HONEYDEW MELON	1/2 cup	30
JICAMA	2 oz	13
KIWIFRUIT	2 oz	35
LASAGNA		
meat	8 oz	327
vegetable	8 oz	245
LETTUCE		
iceberg	1 cup	7
romaine	1 cup	9
MACARONI AND CHEESE	6 oz	214

Prot. MGS	Carbs. GMS	Sodium MGS	Fiber GMS	Fat GMS	Sat. Fat GMS	Chol. MGS	% Fat Cal.
12.0	14.0	864	na	<1.0	na	22	0%
20.6	0.0	539	na	1.1	0.1	55	11%
1.0	4.0	74	0	1.0	0.0	2	36%
0.0	1.0	<5	na	0.8	na	0	60%
2.0	12.0	95	na	8.0	2.5	4	60%
0.0	2.0	1	1.0	0.0	0.0	0	0%
1.5	16.5	66	na	1.7	1.7	0	18%
7.1	0.7	71	na	5.7	na	242	60%
4.0	0.0	35	0	3.0	1.0	122	61%
3.0	15.0	5	0	1.0	0.0	5	11%
2.0	0.0	54	na	na	na	71	0%
4.0	5.0	100	na	0.0	na	10	0%
5.0	45.0	245	4.0	12.0	6.0	0	30%
0.0	8.0	1	1.0	0.0	0.0	0	0%
3.0	7.4	na	na	18.4	na	0	58%
0.0	2.0	425	0	4.0	1.0	0	86%
48.0	0.0	137	na	3.0	0.7	114	11%
36.0	0.0	103	na	2.0	0.5	86	10%
45.0	36.0	335	1.0	33.0	12.0	142	47%
0.0	8.0	9	1.0	0.0	0.0	0	0%
1.0	3.0	1	0	0.0	0.0	0	0%
1.0	8.0	3	2.0	0.0	0.0	0	0%
21.0	23.0	657	na	13.0	6.0	37	36%
15.0	29.0	553	na	8.0	5.0	19	29%
1.0	1.0	5	1.0	0.0	0.0	0	0%
1.0	1.0	4	1.0	0.0	0.0	0	0%
10.0	22.0	590	na	9.0	5.0	26	38%

Food Name	Serving Size	Total Calories
MARGARINE, whipped	1.5 tbsp	105
MARINARA SAUCE	1 oz	13
MEATBALLS	4 meatballs	157
MILK, low-fat	1 cup	140
MINESTRONE SOUP	4 oz	36
MUSHROOMS, raw	1/4 cup	4
OKRA, breaded, unprepared, approx 3.5 oz	1 serving	105
OLIVES	1 oz	47
ONION, red, raw	2 tbsp	8
ONION RINGS, steak cut, breaded, unprepared, approx 3.5 oz	1 serving	395
PASTA AND NOODLES. See SALAD and individual listings.		
PEACH	1/4 cup	34
PEAS	1/4 cup	31
PEPPER, BELL	2 oz	8
PINEAPPLE	1/2 cup	38
PIZZA, 'Supreme' round, 5-inch pie	6.5 oz	524
POLLACK, breaded	4 oz	140
POTATO, BAKED, pulp only	4 oz	105
POTATO SKINS	2 oz	160
RAVIOLI, CHEESE	4 oz	260
REFRIED BEANS	3 oz	120
RICE PILAF	6 oz	256
ROAST BEEF, sliced	2/3 oz	17
SALAD		
beef, teriyaki, 2 oz	1 serving	49
carrot and raisin, 2 oz	1 serving	130
chicken, Chinese, 2 oz	1 serving	54
four bean, approx 3.5 oz	1 serving	104
fruit, 'Mediterranean Minted' 2 oz	1 serving	29
jicama, spicy, 2 oz	1 serving	16
macaroni and cheddar, approx 3.5 oz	1 serving	185

Prot. MGS	Carbs. GMS	Sodium MGS	Fiber GMS	Fat GMS	Sat. Fat GMS	Chol. MGS	% Fat Cal.
0.0	0.0	146	0	11.7	2.0	0	100%
0.0	3.0	90	0	0.0	0.0	0	0%
9.0	5.0	461	1.0	11.0	5.0	30	63%
10.0	13.0	150	na	5.0	2.8	10	32%
1.0	7.0	443	2.0	0.0	0.0	1	0%
0.0	1.0	1	0	0.0	0.0	0	0%
3.3	24.4	503	na	0.5	0.0	<1	4%
1.0	1.0	181	1.0	4.0	1.0	0	77%
0.0	2.0	1	0	0.0	0.0	0	0%
4.8	39.0	558	na	24.4	0.0	0	56%
0.0	9.0	3	1.0	0.0	0.0	0	0%
2.0	6.0	35	2.0	0.0	0.0	0	0%
1.0	2.0	1	1.0	0.0	0.0	0	0%
0.0	10.0	1	1.0	0.0	0.0	0	0%
18.0	51.8	1057	na	27.1	na	14	47%
14.0	18.0	280	na	1.0	na	35	6%
2.0	24.0	6	2.0	0.0	0.0	0	0%
2.0	22.0	463	3.0	8.0	1.0	0	45%
10.0	47.0	270	na	4.0	2.0	20	14%
5.0	16.0	320	na	4.0	1.5	2	30%
4.0	47.0	866	1.0	5.0	1.0	0	18%
3.3	0.3	276	na	0.3	0.1	8	16%
4.0	5.0	136	1.0	2.0	1.0	7	37%
1.0	10.0	104	1.0	10.0	2.0	10	69%
4.0	6.0	119	1.0	2.0	0.0	10	33%
2.6	18.8	226	na	2.5	0.4	0	22%
1.0	7.0	11	0	0.0	0.0	0	0%
0.0	4.0	28	0	0.0	0.0	0	0%
3.2	15.7	476	na	12.5	3.8	14	61%

Food Name	Serving Size	Total Calories
'Mexican Fiesta' 2 oz	1 serving	54
pasta, Italian, approx 3.5 oz	1 serving	90
pasta, Oriental, approx 3.5 oz	1 serving	114
pasta, seafood Louis, 2 oz	1 serving	64
pasta, shell, approx 3.5 oz	1 serving	112
pasta, tuna, 2 oz	1 serving	133
pasta, tuna, chunky, approx 3.5 oz	1 serving	186
potato, German, approx 3.5 oz	1 serving	115
potato, old fashioned, approx 3.5 oz	1 serving	150
potato, red herb, approx 3.5 oz	1 serving	213
potato and egg, approx 3.5 oz	1 serving	140
seafood, 2 oz	1 serving	56
tuna, approx 3.5 oz	1 serving	353
SALAD DRESSING		
blue cheese	1 oz	111
honey mustard	1 oz	160
hot bacon	1 tbsp	40
Italian, lite	1 oz	14
Japanese rice vinegar, fat-free	1 oz	10
Malibu	1 tbsp	100
Parmesan Italian	1 oz	100
ranch	1 oz	120
ranch, reduced calorie	1 oz	90
sour	2 tbsp	60
Thousand Island	1 oz	143
SALMON		
8-oz portion	1 serving	247
3.5-oz portion	1 serving	125
SALSA	1 oz	7
SAUCE		
buttery dipping	1.5 oz	330
hibachi	1.5 oz	57
Malibu	1.5 oz	283

Prot. MGS	Carbs. GMS	Sodium MGS	Fiber GMS	Fat GMS	Sat. Fat GMS	Chol. MGS	% Fat Cal.
2.0	10.0	99	1.0	1.0	0.0	0	17%
3.9	18.3	352	na	0.6	0.1	0	6%
3.7	22.6	781	na	1.6	0.2	<1	13%
3.0	9.0	139	1.0	2.0	0.0	17	28%
3.2	19.4	591	na	2.7	0.5	1	22%
6.0	6.0	188	0	10.0	1.0	10	68%
6.0	14.5	365	na	11.0	2.8	17	53%
2.2	23.1	666	na	2.0	0.5	1	16%
1.6	17.0	416	na	8.7	1.3	23	52%
1.5	15.4	437	na	16.2	2.4	15	68%
1.6	16.0	340	na	7.8	1.2	28	50%
3.0	4.0	255	0	3.0	1.0	7	48%
8.1	7.3	296	na	32.9	5.0	44	84%
1.0	1.0	168	0	12.0	4.0	8	97%
0.0	4.0	110	0	16.0	2.0	10	90%
0.0	5.8	90	na	2.0	na	na	45%
0.0	2.0	350	0	0.0	0.0	0	0%
0.0	2.0	172	0	0.0	0.0	0	0%
0.0	0.0	125	na	11.0	2.0	10	99%
0.0	2.0	450	0	10.0	2.0	0	90%
0.0	2.0	240	0	12.0	2.0	10	90%
0.0	4.0	270	0	8.0	2.0	10	80%
0.0	0.0	30	0	6.0	5.0	0	90%
0.0	3.0	125	0	15.0	2.0	11	94%
32.0	0.0	232	0	12.0	2.0	41	44%
20.0	0.0	50	na	5.0	1.0	70	36%
0.0	2.0	156	0	0.0	0.0	0	0%
0.0	0.0	0	0	36.7	7.0	0	100%
0.0	11.0	707	0	0.0	0.0	0	0%
0.0	0.0	354	0	31.0	6.0	28	99%

Food Name	Serving Size	Total Calories
SCALLOP, breaded, approx 30-40	4 oz	160
SHRIMP		
broiled	5 oz	150
scampi	5 oz	143
tempura batter, approx 21-25	3 oz	155
SIRLOIN STEAK		
9.25-oz size	1 serving	655
6.25-oz size	1 serving	447
top sirloin	1 oz	55
SPAGHETTI	2 oz	80
SPINACH, raw	1/2 cup	6
STRAWBERRIES	1/2 cup	22
STRAWBERRY TOPPING	1 oz	70
STRIP STEAK, New York, 12 oz	1 serving	600
SWORDFISH	8 oz	315
TACO SHELL	1 shell	50
TARTAR SAUCE	1.5 oz	170
TOMATO, cherry	1/4 cup	12
TUNA, yellowfin, approx 3.5 oz	1 serving	125
TURKEY HAM	1 oz	62
VEGETABLE SIRLION SOUP	4 oz	60
VEGETABLE SOUP, vegetarian	6 oz	50
WATERMELON	1/2 cup	26
WHIPPED TOPPING	1 tbsp	12
YOGURT, FROZEN		
chocolate, soft-serve	4 oz	136
vanilla, soft-serve	4 oz	136
ZUCCHINI		
beer-battered, unprepared, approx 3.5 oz	1 serving	205
raw	1/4 cup	5

Prot. MGS	Carbs. GMS	Sodium MGS	Fiber GMS	Fat GMS	Sat. Fat GMS	Chol. MGS	% Fat Cal.
14.0	24.0	393	na	1.0	na	18	6%
23.0	0.0	377	0	6.0	1.0	218	36%
27.0	0.0	386	0	3.0	1.0	150	19%
10.0	13.0	442	na	8.0	3.0	74	46%
80.0	0.0	309	0	35.0	18.0	175	48%
55.0	0.0	245	0	34.0	12.0	120	68%
8.6	na	19	na	2.0	0.7	25	33%
3.0	16.0	1	1.0	0.0	0.0	0	0%
1.0	1.0	22	1.0	0.0	0.0	0	0%
0.0	5.0	1	2.0	0.0	0.0	0	0%
0.0	18.0	5	0	0.0	0.0	0	0%
70.0	5.0	200	na	35.0	na	180	53%
45.0	0.0	331	0	14.0	3.0	89	40%
1.0	7.0	20	1.0	2.0	0.0	0	36%
0.0	6.0	453	0	17.0	3.0	14	90%
0.0	3.0	5	1.0	0.0	0.0	0	0%
15.0	0.0	50	na	4.0	1.0	65	29%
4.0	0.0	376	0	5.0	2.0	19	73%
6.0	6.0	364	0	2.0	1.0	10	30%
2.0	6.0	630	na	1.0	0.2	0	18%
0.0	6.0	2	0	0.0	0.0	0	0%
0.0	1.0	0	0	1.0	1.0	0	75%
1.0	24.0	100	0	4.0	4.0	0	26%
1.0	24.0	100	0	4.0	4.0	0	26%
2.8	23.1	229	na	11.8	0.0	<1	52%
0.0	1.0	1	1.0	0.0	0.0	0	0%

Food Name	Serving Size	Total Calories

SKIPPER'S

Food Name	Serving Size	Total Calories
BARBECUE SAUCE	1 tbsp	25
CHICKEN ENTRÉE		
tenderloin strips, 5 pieces, w/fries	1 serving	793
3 pieces, w/small green salad, 'Lite Catch'	1 serving	305
CHICKEN SANDWICH, 'Create A Catch'	1 serving	606
CHICKEN STRIPS, 'Create A Catch'	1 serving	82
CHOWDER		
'Alder Smoked Salmon'	6 oz	166
clam, 'Create A Catch' cup	1 serving	100
clam, 'Create A Catch' pint	1 serving	200
CLAM ENTRÉE, strips, w/fries 'Basket'	1 serving	1003
COCKTAIL SAUCE	1 tbsp	20
COD ENTRÉE		
thick cut, 3 pieces, w/fries	1 serving	665
thick cut, 4 pieces, w/fries	1 serving	759
thick cut, 5 pieces, w/fries	1 serving	853
COLESLAW, 'Create A Catch' 5 oz . . .	1 serving	289
COMBINATION ENTRÉE		
chicken strips, 1 piece fish, and fries . .	1 serving	805
chicken strips, shrimp, and fries	1 serving	800
clam strips, 1 piece fish, and fries, 'Combos'	1 serving	868
jumbo shrimp, 1 piece fish, and fries, 'Combos'	1 serving	720
1 piece fish, 2 pieces chicken, and small green salad, 'Lite Catch'	1 serving	399
shrimp, 1 piece fish, and fries, 'Combos'	1 serving	728
oysters, 1 piece fish, and fries, 'Combos'	1 serving	885

Prot. MGS	Carbs. GMS	Sodium MGS	Fiber GMS	Fat GMS	Sat. Fat GMS	Chol. MGS	% Fat Cal.
0.0	5.0	226	na	1.0	na	0	36%
44.0	69.0	798	(mq)	38.0	(mq)	77	43%
26.0	17.0	673	(mq)	15.0	(mq)	58	44%
31.0	44.0	976	(mq)	32.0	(mq)	82	48%
8.0	4.0	150	(mq)	4.0	(mq)	15	44%
13.0	14.0	73	na	7.0	na	na	38%
3.0	14.0	525	(mq)	3.5	(mq)	12	32%
5.0	19.0	1050	(mq)	7.0	(mq)	24	32%
22.0	90.0	569	(mq)	70.0	(mq)	14	63%
0.0	5.0	216	na	0.0	0.0	0	0%
27.0	68.0	1054	(mq)	32.0	(mq)	38	43%
34.0	74.0	1388	(mq)	36.0	(mq)	50	43%
42.0	80.0	1723	(mq)	41.0	(mq)	62	43%
2.0	10.0	329	(mq)	27.0	(mq)	50	84%
80.0	72.0	858	(mq)	40.0	(mq)	100	45%
36.0	77.0	1036	(mq)	39.0	(mq)	97	44%
25.0	81.0	667	(mq)	54.0	(mq)	61	56%
24.0	75.0	1268	(mq)	36.0	(mq)	91	45%
29.0	24.0	880	(mq)	21.0	(mq)	96	47%
24.0	77.0	943	(mq)	37.0	(mq)	105	46%
25.0	95.0	809	(mq)	44.0	(mq)	80	45%

Food Name	Serving Size	Total Calories
FISH ENTRÉE. See also individual listings.		
1 fish fillet, w/fries	1 serving	558
2 fish fillets, w/fries	1 serving	733
2 fish fillets, w/small green salad, 'Lite Catch'	1 serving	409
3 fish fillets, w/fries	1 serving	908
FISH FILLET, 'Create A Catch'	1 serving	175
FISH SANDWICH		
'Create A Catch'	1 serving	524
double, 'Create A Catch'	1 serving	698
FRENCH FRIES, 'Create A Catch'	1 serving	383
GELATIN DESSERT, Jell-O, 'Create A Catch'	1 serving	55
MILK, low-fat	12 oz	181
OYSTER ENTRÉE, w/fries, 'Basket'	1 serving	1038
POTATO, BAKED	1 serving	145
ROOT BEER FLOAT	1 serving	302
SALAD		
green, small, 'Lite Catch'	1 serving	59
shrimp and seafood	1 serving	167
side order	1 serving	24
SALAD DRESSING		
blue cheese, premium	1 pouch	222
Italian, gourmet	1 pouch	140
Italian, low-calorie	1 pouch	17
ranch house	1 pouch	188
Thousand Island	1 pouch	160
SALMON, baked	4.4 oz	270
SEAFOOD ENTRÉE, w/fries, 'Skipper's Platter Basket'	1 serving	1038
SHRIMP ENTRÉE		
jumbo, w/fries, 'Basket'	1 serving	707
original, w/fries, 'Basket'	1 serving	723

Prot. MGS	Carbs. GMS	Sodium MGS	Fiber GMS	Fat GMS	Sat. Fat GMS	Chol. MGS	% Fat Cal.
17.0	51.0	408	(mq)	28.0	(mq)	55	45%
28.0	71.0	765	(mq)	38.0	(mq)	108	47%
25.0	27.0	937	(mq)	23.0	(mq)	119	51%
39.0	82.0	1122	(mq)	48.0	(mq)	160	48%
11.0	11.0	357	(mq)	10.0	(mq)	53	51%
19.0	43.0	1191	(mq)	33.0	(mq)	86	57%
30.0	54.0	1548	(mq)	73.0	(mq)	139	94%
6.0	50.0	51	(mq)	18.0	(mq)	2	42%
1.0	12.0	35	0	0.0	0.0	0	0%
15.0	32.0	225	na	10.0	na	0	50%
28.0	118.0	853	(mq)	51.0	(mq)	52	44%
4.0	32.0	6	na	0.0	na	0	0%
3.0	33.0	66	na	10.0	(mq)	10	30%
3.0	6.0	223	(mq)	3.0	(mq)	13	46%
23.0	15.0	657	na	3.0	na	80	16%
0.0	4.0	8	na	0.0	na	0	0%
1.0	4.0	240	na	23.0	(mq)	8	93%
0.0	2.0	200	na	15.0	(mq)	0	96%
0.0	2.0	680	na	1.0	na	0	53%
1.0	2.0	302	na	20.0	(mq)	0	96%
0.0	8.0	415	na	14.0	(mq)	6	79%
39.0	1.0	504	na	11.0	na	70	37%
32.0	97.0	1202	(mq)	63.0	(mq)	111	55%
20.0	79.0	911	(mq)	35.0	(mq)	73	45%
20.0	82.0	1121	(mq)	36.0	(mq)	102	45%

Food Name	Serving Size	Total Calories
w/seafood salad, 'Lite Catch'	1 serving	167
TARTAR SAUCE	1 tbsp	65

SONIC

Food Name	Serving Size	Total Calories
BACON, LETTUCE, AND TOMATO SANDWICH 'B-L-T'	1 sandwich	327
CHEESE SANDWICH, grilled	1 sandwich	288
CHEESEBURGER		
bacon	1 serving	548
double meat and cheese, w/mayonnaise, 'Super Sonic'	1 serving	730
double meat and cheese, w/mustard, 'Super Sonic'	1 serving	644
jalapeño, double meat, and cheese ...	1 serving	638
mini	1 serving	281
#2 cheeseburger	1 serving	70
CHICKEN SANDWICH		
....	1 serving	319
breaded	1 serving	455
grilled	1 serving	265
grilled, w/o dressing	1 serving	215
CHILI PIE	1 serving	327
FISH SANDWICH	1 serving	277
FRENCH FRIES		
large order	1 serving	315
large order, w/cheese	1 serving	420
regular order	1 serving	233
HAMBURGER		
hickory	1 serving	314
mini	1 serving	246
HOT DOG		
corn dog	1 serving	280

Prot. MGS	Carbs. GMS	Sodium MGS	Fiber GMS	Fat GMS	Sat. Fat GMS	Chol. MGS	% Fat Cal.
23.0	15.0	657	(mq)	3.0	(mq)	80	16%
0.0	0.0	102	na	7.0	(mq)	4	97%
8.3	26.5	600	na	19.3	na	9	53%
11.9	25.3	841	na	17.0	na	36	53%
27.7	23.0	839	na	38.6	na	87	63%
43.8	23.9	1023	na	51.5	na	144	63%
43.8	23.9	1128	na	40.7	na	136	57%
43.6	21.6	1358	na	40.6	na	136	57%
16.5	20.3	644	na	14.4	na	45	46%
4.4	0.3	267	na	5.8	na	18	75%
21.0	41.0	890	na	9.0	na	47	25%
22.7	36.4	755	na	24.7	na	42	49%
21.0	23.0	716	na	10.0	na	63	34%
21.0	23.3	716	na	4.3	na	63	18%
11.5	20.1	313	na	22.6	na	28	62%
17.0	38.0	655	na	7.0	na	6	23%
4.5	49.5	67	na	11.2	na	11	32%
10.5	50.5	468	na	20.2	na	38	43%
3.0	37.0	50	na	8.0	na	8	31%
19.9	23.3	459	na	15.7	na	50	45%
14.4	20.1	510	na	11.5	na	36	42%
7.0	30.0	700	na	15.0	na	35	48%

Food Name	Serving Size	Total Calories
extra long, 'Cheese Coney'	1 serving	635
extra long, w/onions, 'Cheese Coney' .	1 serving	640
#2 hot dog	1 serving	323
regular	1 serving	258
regular, 'Cheese Coney'	1 serving	358
regular, w/onions, 'Cheese Coney' ...	1 serving	361
ONION RINGS		
large order	1 serving	577
regular order	1 serving	404
POTATO NUGGETS		
Tater Tots	1 serving	150
Tater Tots, w/cheese	1 serving	220
STEAK SANDWICH, breaded	1 serving	631

SPAGHETTI WAREHOUSE

MINESTRONE SOUP	1 serving	56
SPAGHETTI W/MARINARA SAUCE		
dinner portion	1 serving	403
lunch portion	1 serving	298
SPAGHETTI W/TOMATO SAUCE		
dinner portion	1 serving	410
lunch portion	1 serving	301

STEAK 'N SHAKE

APPLE DANISH	1 pastry	391
BAKED BEANS	1 serving	173
BREAKFAST SANDWICH		
egg	1 serving	275
ham, w/egg	1 serving	434
BROWNIE	1 brownie	258
CHEESE SANDWICH, toasted	1 serving	250

Prot. MGS	Carbs. GMS	Sodium MGS	Fiber GMS	Fat GMS	Sat. Fat GMS	Chol. MGS	% Fat Cal.
24.4	45.4	632	na	39.0	na	65	55%
25.0	47.0	632	na	39.2	na	65	55%
19.9	23.3	549	na	15.7	na	50	44%
8.2	21.3	241	na	15.3	na	23	53%
14.0	23.1	341	na	23.3	na	40	59%
14.0	23.7	341	na	23.3	na	40	58%
7.6	54.1	532	na	37.8	na	na	59%
5.3	37.9	372	na	26.5	na	na	59%
2.0	19.0	330	na	7.0	na	10	42%
6.0	19.3	569	na	13.0	na	28	53%
18.6	46.4	1047	na	41.6	na	50	59%
3.0	8.0	155	2.0	1.0	na	3	16%
13.0	75.0	303	5.0	5.0	na	0	11%
10.0	56.0	210	4.0	4.0	na	0	12%
13.0	76.0	454	6.0	5.0	na	0	11%
10.0	56.0	303	4.0	3.0	na	0	9%
6.0	35.0	352	na	24.0	na	na	55%
9.0	27.0	656	na	4.0	na	na	21%
12.0	33.0	490	na	10.0	na	na	33%
36.0	33.0	1850	na	17.0	na	na	35%
3.0	39.0	165	na	12.0	na	na	42%
9.0	24.0	606	na	13.0	na	na	47%

Food Name	Serving Size	Total Calories
CHEESEBURGER		
steakburger	1 serving	353
steakburger, super	1 serving	451
steakburger, triple	1 serving	626
CHEESECAKE		
plain	1 serving	368
w/strawberries	1 serving	386
CHILI		
'Chili Mac' w/4 saltines	1 serving	310
'Chili 3 Ways' w/4 saltines	1 serving	411
w/oyster crackers	1 serving	337
COTTAGE CHEESE	1/2 cup	93
DESSERT		
'Coca-Cola Float'	1 serving	514
'Lemon Float'	1 serving	555
'Lemon Freeze'	1 serving	548
'Orange Float'	1 serving	502
'Orange Freeze'	1 serving	516
'Root Beer Float'	1 serving	529
FRENCH FRIES	1 serving	211
HAM SANDWICH, baked	1 serving	451
HAMBURGER		
steakburger	1 serving	277
steakburger, super	1 serving	375
steakburger, triple	1 serving	474
HOT CHOCOLATE	1 serving	686
ICE CREAM, vanilla	1 serving	213
MILKSHAKE		
chocolate	1 serving	608
strawberry	1 serving	648
vanilla	1 serving	619
PIE		
apple	1 serving	407

Prot. MGS	Carbs. GMS	Sodium MGS	Fiber GMS	Fat GMS	Sat. Fat GMS	Chol. MGS	% Fat Cal.
23.0	33.0	658	na	13.0	na	na	33%
35.0	33.0	680	na	18.0	na	na	36%
52.0	34.0	934	na	30.0	na	na	43%
7.0	61.0	294	na	11.0	na	na	27%
7.0	65.0	294	na	11.0	na	na	26%
15.0	34.0	1301	na	12.0	na	na	35%
19.0	45.0	1734	na	16.0	na	na	35%
16.0	37.0	1157	na	14.0	na	na	37%
12.0	3.0	198	na	4.0	na	na	39%
16.0	76.0	230	na	17.0	na	na	30%
18.0	82.0	248	na	19.0	na	na	31%
15.0	69.0	213	na	25.0	na	na	41%
16.0	74.0	224	na	17.0	na	na	30%
14.0	63.0	198	na	24.0	na	na	42%
17.0	78.0	237	na	17.0	na	na	29%
3.0	28.0	297	na	10.0	na	na	43%
29.0	37.0	1858	na	22.0	na	na	44%
18.0	33.0	425	na	7.0	na	na	23%
30.0	33.0	447	na	12.0	na	na	29%
43.0	33.0	468	na	17.0	na	na	32%
17.0	129.0	669	na	19.0	na	na	25%
1.0	23.0	70	na	12.0	na	na	51%
13.0	57.0	178	na	38.0	na	na	56%
16.0	62.0	191	na	40.0	na	na	56%
13.0	58.0	181	na	38.0	na	na	55%
4.0	61.0	479	na	18.0	na	na	40%

Food Name	Serving Size	Total Calories
apple 'À la mode'	1 serving	549
cherry	1 serving	334
cherry 'À la mode'	1 serving	476
SALAD		
chef's	1 serving	313
lettuce and tomato, w/1 oz Thousand Island dressing	1 serving	168
STEAK ENTRÉE, platter, low-calorie	1 serving	293
SUNDAE		
fudge brownie	1 serving	645
hot fudge nut	1 serving	530
strawberry	1 serving	330

SUBWAY

Food Name	Serving Size	Total Calories
SALAD		
chef's, small	1 serving	189
garden, large	1 serving	46
ham, small	1 serving	170
roast beef, small	1 serving	185
seafood and crab, small	1 serving	198
tuna, small	1 serving	212
turkey, small	1 serving	167
SALAD DRESSING, Italian, lite	4 tbsp	23
SUBMARINE SANDWICH		
club, Italian, 12-inch	1 sandwich	693
club, Italian, on honey wheat roll, 12-inch	1 sandwich	722
ham, 6-inch	1 sandwich	360
ham and cheese, Italian, 12-inch	1 sandwich	643
ham and cheese, on honey wheat roll, 12-inch	1 sandwich	673
Italian cold cut combo, 12-inch	1 sandwich	853

Prot. MGS	Carbs. GMS	Sodium MGS	Fiber GMS	Fat GMS	Sat. Fat GMS	Chol. MGS	% Fat Cal.
4.0	76.0	525	na	25.0	na	na	41%
6.0	48.0	268	na	14.0	na	na	38%
6.0	63.0	314	na	22.0	na	na	42%
41.0	6.0	1582	na	18.0	na	na	52%
1.0	7.0	223	na	15.0	na	na	80%
37.0	3.0	242	na	14.0	na	na	43%
7.0	81.0	262	na	35.0	na	na	49%
5.0	51.0	121	na	34.0	na	na	58%
2.0	29.0	81	na	22.0	na	na	60%
19.0	6.0	479	na	10.0	na	na	48%
2.0	10.0	634	na	0.0	na	0	0%
14.0	6.0	479	na	10.0	na	na	53%
18.0	6.0	479	na	10.0	na	na	49%
12.0	13.0	946	na	11.0	na	na	50%
20.0	8.0	545	na	12.0	na	na	51%
15.0	4.0	479	na	9.0	na	na	49%
1.0	4.0	952	na	<1.0	na	<1	0%
46.0	83.0	2716	na	22.0	na	84	29%
47.0	89.0	2776	na	23.0	na	84	29%
20.0	45.0	839	na	11.0	na	na	28%
38.0	81.0	1709	na	18.0	na	73	25%
39.0	86.0	2508	na	22.0	na	73	29%
46.0	83.0	2218	na	40.0	na	166	42%

Food Name	Serving Size	Total Calories
Italian cold cut combo, on honey wheat roll, 12-inch	1 sandwich	882
meatball, 6-inch	1 sandwich	429
meatball, Italian, 12-inch	1 sandwich	917
meatball, on honey wheat roll, 12-inch	1 sandwich	947
roast beef, 6-inch	1 sandwich	375
roast beef, Italian, 12-inch	1 sandwich	689
roast beef, on honey wheat roll, 12-inch	1 sandwich	717
seafood and crab, 6-inch	1 sandwich	388
steak, 6-inch	1 sandwich	423
steak and cheese, Italian, 12-inch	1 sandwich	765
steak and cheese, on honey wheat roll, 12-inch	1 sandwich	711
subway club, 6-inch	1 sandwich	379
tuna, 6-inch	1 sandwich	402
turkey, 6-inch	1 sandwich	357
turkey breast, Italian, 12-inch	1 sandwich	645
turkey breast, on honey wheat roll, 12-inch	1 sandwich	674
veggies and cheese, Italian, 12-inch	1 sandwich	535

SWENSEN'S

ICE CREAM

'Almond Praline Delight' low-fat	1/2 cup	130
'Caramel Apple Crisp' low-fat	1/2 cup	130
'Caramel Turtle Fudge' light	1 serving	120
'Caramel Turtle Fudge' low-fat	1/2 cup	140
'Chocolate Chocolate Chip Cheesecake' low-fat	1/2 cup	130
'Chocolate Fudge Brownie' low-fat	1/2 cup	120

Prot. MGS	Carbs. GMS	Sodium MGS	Fiber GMS	Fat GMS	Sat. Fat GMS	Chol. MGS	% Fat Cal.
48.0	88.0	2278	na	41.0	na	166	42%
26.0	45.0	876	na	16.0	na	na	34%
42.0	96.0	2022	na	44.0	na	88	43%
44.0	101.0	2082	na	45.0	na	88	43%
24.0	45.0	839	na	11.0	na	na	26%
42.0	84.0	2287	na	23.0	na	75	30%
41.0	89.0	2347	na	24.0	na	75	30%
18.0	52.0	1306	na	12.0	na	na	28%
28.0	46.0	883	na	14.0	na	na	30%
43.0	83.0	1556	na	32.0	na	82	38%
41.0	89.0	1615	na	33.0	na	82	42%
25.0	45.0	839	na	11.0	na	na	26%
26.0	45.0	905	na	13.0	na	na	29%
21.0	46.0	839	na	10.0	na	na	25%
40.0	83.0	2459	na	19.0	na	67	27%
42.0	88.0	2520	na	20.0	na	67	27%
20.0	81.0	1076	na	17.0	na	19	29%
3.0	25.0	85	0	2.0	1.0	5	14%
3.0	26.0	75	0	1.0	0.5	<5	7%
3.0	18.0	50	na	4.0	na	10	30%
3.0	26.0	70	0	2.5	1.0	5	16%
3.0	26.0	80	0	2.5	1.0	<5	17%
3.0	24.0	70	0	2.5	1.0	<5	19%

Food Name	Serving Size	Total Calories
'Cookies 'n' Cream' light	1 serving	130
'Cookies 'n' Cream' low-fat	1/2 cup	130
'Vanilla' light	1 serving	110
YOGURT, FROZEN		
'Black Forest Cake'	1 serving	95
'Black Forest Cake' low-fat	1/2 cup	110
'Blueberry 'n' Cream' gourmet, sugar-free	1 serving	110
'Butter Pecan' low-fat	1/2 cup	120
'Cherry' nonfat	1/2 cup	90
'Chocolate Raspberry Truffle' gourmet, sugar-free	1 serving	130
'Coconut Pineapple'	1 serving	120
'Hazelnut Amaretto' low-fat	1/2 cup	120
'Mocha Chip' low-fat	1/2 cup	110
'Strawberry Banana 'n' Cream' nonfat	1/2 cup	90
'Triple Chocolate' low-fat	1/2 cup	120
'Triple Chocolate' nonfat	1 serving	100
'Vanilla' nonfat	1/2 cup	90
'Vanilla Swiss Almond' gourmet, sugar-free	1 serving	140

SWISS CHALET

CAKE		
Black Forest	1 piece	278
fudge nut	1 piece	346
CHICKEN	1/2 chicken	634
CHICKEN SALAD	1 serving	500
CHICKEN SANDWICH		
cold	1 sandwich	360
hot	1 sandwich	310
CHICKEN SOUP, 'Chalet'	1 serving	97
COLESLAW, 'Chalet'	1 serving	56

Prot. MGS	Carbs. GMS	Sodium MGS	Fiber GMS	Fat GMS	Sat. Fat GMS	Chol. MGS	% Fat Cal.
3.0	20.0	60	na	4.0	na	10	28%
3.0	25.0	80	0	2.5	0.5	<5	17%
3.0	15.0	50	na	4.0	na	10	33%
3.0	21.0	130	na	1.0	na	5	9%
4.0	22.0	55	1.0	1.5	1.0	0	12%
3.0	17.0	90	na	4.0	na	10	33%
4.0	20.0	55	0	3.0	0.5	<5	23%
3.0	20.0	45	0	0.0	0.0	0	0%
3.0	18.0	80	na	5.0	na	8	35%
4.0	26.0	65	na	1.0	na	5	8%
4.0	20.0	50	0	3.0	0.0	0	23%
4.0	22.0	50	0	1.5	1.0	0	12%
3.0	20.0	45	0	0.0	0.0	0	0%
4.0	24.0	50	1.0	1.5	1.0	0	11%
4.0	21.0	65	na	0.0	0.0	0	0%
3.0	20.0	60	0	0.0	0.0	0	0%
4.0	15.0	100	na	7.0	na	10	45%
3.0	36.0	na	na	14.0	na	na	45%
4.0	48.0	na	na	16.0	na	na	42%
72.0	1.0	na	na	38.0	na	na	54%
42.0	23.0	na	na	42.0	na	na	76%
33.0	42.0	na	na	5.0	na	na	13%
30.0	30.0	na	na	6.0	na	na	17%
9.0	11.0	na	na	2.0	na	na	19%
2.0	10.0	na	na	1.0	na	na	16%

Food Name	Serving Size	Total Calories
FRENCH FRIES	1 serving	478
GRAVY, sandwich	1 serving	35
ICE CREAM, vanilla	1 serving	195
PASTRY, chocolate éclair	1 serving	205
PIE		
apple	1 serving	394
coconut	1 serving	292
POTATO, BAKED	1 serving	227
ROLL	1 roll	116

TACO BELL

BURRITO		
bean	7.3 oz	447
beef	7.3 oz	493
beef, double, 'Supreme'	1 serving	451
beef, 'MexiMelt'	3.7 oz	266
'Cheesarito'	1 serving	312
chicken	6 oz	334
chicken, 'MexiMelt'	3.8 oz	257
combination	7 oz	407
'Light' bean	7.07 oz	330
'Light' burrito supreme	8.86 oz	350
'Light' 7-layer	9.53 oz	440
'Supreme'	9 oz	503
CHEESE SAUCE, nacho	2 oz	103
FAJITA, chicken	1 serving	226
FAJITA TACO		
steak	1 serving	235
steak, w/guacamole	1 serving	269
steak, w/sour cream	1 serving	281
GREEN SAUCE	1 oz	4
GUACAMOLE	.75 oz	34

Prot. MGS	Carbs. GMS	Sodium MGS	Fiber GMS	Fat GMS	Sat. Fat GMS	Chol. MGS	% Fat Cal.
10.0	57.0	na	na	24.0	na	na	45%
1.0	5.0	na	na	1.0	na	na	26%
3.0	16.0	na	na	14.0	na	na	65%
2.0	27.0	na	na	10.0	na	na	44%
3.0	45.0	na	na	23.0	na	na	53%
2.0	40.0	na	na	14.0	na	na	43%
8.0	52.0	na	na	tr	na	na	0%
3.0	24.0	na	na	1.0	na	na	8%
15.0	63.0	1148	(mq)	14.0	4.0	9	28%
25.0	48.0	1311	(mq)	21.0	8.0	57	38%
23.0	40.0	928	na	22.0	10.0	59	44%
13.0	19.0	689	(mq)	15.0	8.0	38	51%
12.0	37.0	451	na	13.0	7.0	29	38%
17.0	38.0	880	(mq)	12.0	4.0	52	32%
14.0	19.0	779	(mq)	15.0	7.0	48	53%
18.0	46.0	1136	(mq)	16.0	5.0	33	35%
14.0	55.0	na	na	6.0	na	5	18%
20.0	50.0	na	na	8.0	na	58	20%
19.0	67.0	na	na	9.0	na	5	18%
20.0	55.0	1181	(mq)	22.0	8.0	33	39%
4.0	5.0	393	0	8.0	3.0	9	70%
14.0	20.0	619	na	10.0	4.0	44	40%
15.0	20.0	507	na	11.0	5.0	14	42%
15.0	23.0	620	na	13.0	5.0	14	43%
15.0	21.0	507	na	15.0	7.0	14	48%
0.0	1.0	136	na	0.0	0.0	0	0%
1.0	3.0	113	(mq)	2.0	0.0	0	53%

Food Name	Serving Size	Total Calories
NACHOS		
'Nachos Bellgrande'	10.1 oz	649
'Nachos Supreme'	5.1 oz	367
regular	3.7 oz	346
PASTRY, 'Cinnamon Twists'	1.2 oz	171
PEPPER, JALAPEÑO	3.5 oz	20
PINTO BEANS, w/cheese and red sauce	4.5 oz	190
PIZZA, Mexican	7.9 oz	575
RED SAUCE	1 oz	10
RELISH, 'Pico de Gallo'	.7 oz	6
SALAD		
seafood, w/ranch dressing	1 serving	884
seafood, w/o dressing	1 serving	648
seafood, w/o dressing, w/o shell	1 serving	217
taco, 21 oz	1 serving	905
taco, w/ranch dressing	1 serving	1167
taco, w/o beans	1 serving	822
taco, w/o salsa	1 serving	931
taco, w/o shell, 18.3 oz	1 serving	484
SALAD DRESSING, ranch	2.6 oz	236
SALSA	.34 oz	18
SOUR CREAM	.75 oz	46
TACO		
'Bellgrande'	5.7 oz	335
chicken	3 oz	171
chicken, soft	3.8 oz	213
'Light' soft taco	3.54 oz	180
'Light' soft taco supreme	4.57 oz	200
'Light' taco	2.79 oz	140
'Light' taco salad w/chips	19.11 oz	680
'Light' taco salad w/o chips	16.57 oz	330
'Light' taco supreme	3.79 oz	160
platter, light	1 serving	1062

Prot. MGS	Carbs. GMS	Sodium MGS	Fiber GMS	Fat GMS	Sat. Fat GMS	Chol. MGS	% Fat Cal.
22.0	61.0	997	(mq)	35.0	12.0	36	49%
12.0	41.0	471	(mq)	27.0	5.0	18	66%
7.0	37.0	399	(mq)	18.0	6.0	9	47%
2.0	24.0	234	(mq)	8.0	3.0	0	42%
1.0	4.0	1370	(mq)	0.0	0.0	0	0%
9.0	19.0	642	(mq)	9.0	4.0	16	43%
21.0	40.0	1031	(mq)	37.0	11.0	52	58%
0.0	2.0	261	na	0.0	0.0	0	0%
0.0	1.0	66	na	0.0	0.0	0	0%
25.0	49.0	1489	na	66.0	34.0	117	67%
24.0	47.0	917	na	42.0	30.0	82	58%
18.0	12.0	693	na	11.0	6.0	81	46%
34.0	55.0	910	(mq)	61.0	19.0	80	61%
37.0	61.0	1959	na	87.0	45.0	121	67%
31.0	47.0	1368	na	57.0	38.0	81	62%
35.0	60.0	1387	na	62.0	40.0	85	60%
28.0	22.0	680	(mq)	31.0	14.0	80	58%
2.0	1.0	571	(mq)	25.0	5.0	35	95%
1.0	4.0	376	na	0.0	0.0	0	0%
1.0	1.0	0	0	4.0	2.0	31	78%
18.0	18.0	472	(mq)	23.0	11.0	56	62%
12.0	11.0	337	(mq)	9.0	3.0	52	47%
14.0	19.0	615	(mq)	10.0	4.0	52	42%
13.0	19.0	na	na	5.0	na	25	27%
14.0	23.0	na	na	5.0	na	25	25%
11.0	11.0	na	na	5.0	na	20	36%
35.0	81.0	na	na	25.0	na	50	34%
30.0	35.0	na	na	9.0	na	50	24%
13.0	14.0	na	na	5.0	na	20	31%
38.0	97.0	2068	na	58.0	34.0	82	49%

Food Name	Serving Size	Total Calories
regular	2.75 oz	183
regular, soft	3.25 oz	225
steak, soft	3.5 oz	218
'Supreme'	3.25 oz	230
'Supreme,' soft	4.4 oz	272
TACO SAUCE		
hot	1 pkt	3
regular	1 pkt	2
TOSTADA		
beef	1 serving	322
chicken, w/red sauce	5.8 oz	264
w/red sauce	5.5 oz	243

TACO JOHN'S

BURRITO		
bean	5 oz	249
beef	5 oz	355
chicken, super, w/o sour cream or cheese	1 serving	366
chicken, w/o sour cream or cheese	1 serving	227
combo	5 oz	302
super	8.3 oz	434
super, w/o sour cream or cheese	1 serving	389
w/green chili	12.3 oz	405
w/green chili, w/o sour cream or cheese	1 serving	367
w/Texas chili	12.3 oz	518
CHICKEN SANDWICH, fillet, 'Sierra'	8.5 oz	500
CHILI, Texas	9.5 oz	430
CHIMICHANGA, 'Chimi'	12 oz	487
DANISH, 'Apple Grande'	3 oz	257
ENCHILADA	7 oz	379

Prot. MGS	Carbs. GMS	Sodium MGS	Fiber GMS	Fat GMS	Sat. Fat GMS	Chol. MGS	% Fat Cal.
10.0	11.0	276	(mq)	11.0	5.0	32	54%
12.0	18.0	554	(mq)	12.0	5.0	32	48%
14.0	18.0	456	(mq)	11.0	5.0	30	45%
11.0	12.0	276	(mq)	15.0	8.0	32	59%
13.0	19.0	554	(mq)	16.0	8.0	32	53%
0.0	0.0	82	na	0.0	0.0	0	0%
0.0	0.0	126	na	0.0	0.0	0	0%
15.0	22.0	764	na	20.0	10.0	40	56%
12.0	20.0	454	(mq)	15.0	7.0	37	51%
9.0	27.0	596	(mq)	11.0	4.0	16	41%
10.0	36.0	636	(mq)	6.0	(mq)	na	22%
16.0	25.0	666	(mq)	18.0	(mq)	na	46%
30.0	40.0	844	na	14.0	na	na	34%
27.0	19.0	639	na	10.0	na	na	40%
11.0	30.0	651	(mq)	12.0	(mq)	na	36%
17.0	66.0	1022	(mq)	11.0	(mq)	na	23%
18.0	51.0	856	na	16.0	na	na	37%
18.0	38.0	995	(mq)	24.0	(mq)	na	53%
20.0	40.0	998	na	18.0	na	na	44%
23.0	48.0	746	(mq)	24.0	(mq)	na	42%
31.0	46.0	1493	23.0	21.0	na	41	38%
23.0	35.0	1580	(mq)	22.0	(mq)	(mq)	46%
16.0	54.0	1226	(mq)	19.0	(mq)	(mq)	35%
5.0	44.0	231	(mq)	8.0	(mq)	na	28%
19.0	33.0	431	(mq)	18.0	(mq)	(mq)	43%

Food Name	Serving Size	Total Calories
NACHOS		
regular	4 oz	407
super	11.25 oz	657
PASTRY, 'Churro'	1.2 oz	122
POTATO, BAKED, 'Potato Ole' large	6 oz	414
REFRIED BEANS	9.5 oz	331
RICE, Mexican	1 serving	340
SALAD		
chicken taco, super, w/o dressing or sour cream	1 serving	377
taco, super, 12.3 oz	1 serving	450
taco, super, w/o shell, dressing, or sour cream	1 serving	428
taco, w/o shell, dressing, sour cream, or cheese	1 serving	228
TACO		
chicken, soft shell	1 serving	180
regular	4.3 oz	228
soft shell	5 oz	276
'Taco Bravo' super	8 oz	485
'Taco Bravo' w/o sour cream	1 serving	319
taco burger	6 oz	332
TOSTADA	4.3 oz	228

TACO TIME

BURRITO		
bean, soft	1 serving	547
bean, soft, w/o cheese	1 serving	462
'Casita' w/o sour cream or cheese	1 serving	427
combo, soft	1 serving	550
combo, soft, w/o cheese	1 serving	462
meat, soft, w/o cheese	1 serving	467

Prot. MGS	Carbs. GMS	Sodium MGS	Fiber GMS	Fat GMS	Sat. Fat GMS	Chol. MGS	% Fat Cal.
11.0	42.0	307	(mq)	19.0	(mq)	(mq)	42%
23.0	57.0	857	(mq)	34.0	(mq)	(mq)	47%
1.7	12.0	153	na	7.0	(mq)	na	52%
6.0	96.0	1595	(mq)	6.0	(mq)	na	13%
19.0	79.0	1195	(mq)	6.0	(mq)	na	16%
7.0	59.0	1280	na	8.0	na	na	21%
26.0	56.0	882	na	15.0	na	na	36%
16.0	48.0	880	(mq)	18.0	(mq)	na	36%
21.0	59.0	900	na	20.0	na	na	42%
13.0	30.0	440	na	13.0	na	na	51%
18.0	20.0	490	na	8.0	na	na	40%
11.0	15.0	347	(mq)	13.0	(mq)	(mq)	51%
13.0	23.0	505	(mq)	13.0	(mq)	(mq)	42%
18.0	51.0	1006	(mq)	20.0	(mq)	(mq)	37%
16.0	42.0	658	na	14.0	na	na	39%
14.0	31.0	660	(mq)	14.0	(mq)	(mq)	38%
11.0	15.0	347	(mq)	13.0	(mq)	na	51%
22.0	68.0	1027	na	21.0	na	20	35%
17.0	65.0	895	na	14.0	na	0	27%
23.0	46.0	1243	na	17.0	na	25	36%
30.0	55.0	1227	na	24.0	na	48	39%
17.0	65.0	1095	na	14.0	na	0	27%
32.0	40.0	1295	na	19.0	na	53	37%

Food Name	Serving Size	Total Calories
veggie	1 serving	535
veggie, w/o sour cream	1 serving	502
veggie, w/o sour cream or cheese	1 serving	477
CHEESEBURGER, taco, w/o dressing or cheese	1 serving	397
REFRIED BEANS, 'Refritos' w/o cheese	1 serving	293
RICE, brown, Mexican	1 serving	160
SALAD		
chicken taco, w/o dressing	1 serving	436
chicken taco, w/o dressing or cheese	1 serving	381
side order, w/o dressing or cheese	1 serving	302
taco, w/o dressing	1 serving	347
veggie, w/o dressing or cheese	1 serving	302
SAUCE		
casa	1 oz	40
enchilada	1 oz	14
hot	1 oz	10
ranchero	2 oz	18
TACO		
chicken, soft	1 serving	390
chicken, soft, w/o cheese	1 serving	335
flour, soft, w/o cheese	1 serving	331
TOSTADA, meat, 'Delight' w/o sour cream or cheese	1 serving	410

TCBY

YOGURT, FROZEN, all flavors
Fat-free

giant	31.6 oz	869
super	15.2 oz	418
large	10.5 oz	289
regular	8.2 oz	226

Prot. MGS	Carbs. GMS	Sodium MGS	Fiber GMS	Fat GMS	Sat. Fat GMS	Chol. MGS	% Fat Cal.
21.0	71.0	890	na	20.0	na	20	34%
21.0	71.0	883	na	17.0	na	14	30%
18.0	69.0	798	na	13.0	na	0	25%
20.0	49.0	1071	na	13.0	na	17	29%
11.0	38.0	834	na	11.0	na	0	34%
2.0	28.0	540	na	2.0	na	0	11%
31.0	35.0	521	na	19.0	na	70	39%
29.0	33.0	436	na	15.0	na	56	35%
12.0	36.0	715	na	13.0	na	0	39%
23.0	22.0	720	na	16.0	na	35	41%
12.0	36.0	715	na	13.0	na	0	39%
0.0	10.0	180	na	0.0	0.0	0	0%
0.0	3.0	115	na	0.0	0.0	0	0%
0.0	2.0	120	na	0.0	0.0	0	0%
1.0	3.0	115	na	1.0	na	0	50%
31.0	34.0	322	na	12.0	na	70	28%
29.0	32.0	237	na	8.0	na	56	21%
19.0	34.0	599	na	12.0	na	26	33%
22.0	42.0	916	na	17.0	na	25	37%
32.0	182.0	356	na	0.0	0.0	0	0%
15.0	87.0	171	na	0.0	0.0	0	0%
10.0	60.0	118	na	0.0	0.0	0	0%
8.0	47.0	92	na	0.0	0.0	0	0%

Food Name	Serving Size	Total Calories
small	5.9 oz	162
kiddie	3.2 oz	88
Fat-free, sugar-free		
giant	31.6 oz	632
super	15.2 oz	304
large	10.5 oz	210
regular	8.2 oz	164
small	5.9 oz	118
kiddie	3.2 oz	64
Regular, 96% fat-free		
giant	31.6 oz	1027
super	15.2 oz	494
large	10.5 oz	342
regular	8.2 oz	267
small	5.9 oz	192
kiddie	3.2 oz	104

WENDY'S

Food Name	Serving Size	Total Calories
ALFALFA SPROUTS	1 oz	8
ALFREDO SAUCE	2 oz	35
APPLE TOPPING	1 serving	130
BACON BITS, imitation	1/8 oz	10
BARBECUE SAUCE	1 oz	50
BISCUIT, buttermilk	1 serving	320
BLUEBERRIES	1 tbsp	6
BLUEBERRY TOPPING	1 serving	60
BREADSTICKS		
	1 stick	130
salad bar item	2 sticks	35
BREAKFAST		
bacon	1 strip	30
breakfast sandwich	1 serving	370

Prot. MGS	Carbs. GMS	Sodium MGS	Fiber GMS	Fat GMS	Sat. Fat GMS	Chol. MGS	% Fat Cal.
6.0	34.0	66	na	0.0	0.0	0	0%
3.0	18.0	36	na	0.0	0.0	0	0%
32.0	142.0	316	na	0.0	0.0	0	0%
15.0	68.0	152	na	0.0	0.0	0	0%
10.0	47.0	105	na	0.0	0.0	0	0%
8.0	37.0	82	na	0.0	0.0	0	0%
6.0	27.0	59	na	0.0	0.0	0	0%
3.0	14.0	32	na	0.0	0.0	0	0%
32.0	182.0	474	na	24.0	16.0	79	21%
15.0	87.0	228	na	11.0	8.0	38	20%
10.0	60.0	156	na	8.0	5.0	26	21%
8.0	47.0	126	na	6.0	4.0	20	20%
6.0	34.0	90	na	4.0	3.0	15	19%
3.0	18.0	48	na	2.0	2.0	8	17%
1.0	tr	na	na	tr	na	0	0%
1.0	5.0	300	na	1.0	0.8	tr	26%
tr	32.0	120	na	tr	na	0	0%
1.0	tr	100	na	tr	na	tr	0%
<1.0	11.0	100	na	<1.0	tr	0	0%
5.0	37.0	860	na	17.0	na	tr	48%
1.0	1.0	na	na	tr	na	0	0%
tr	15.0	65	na	tr	na	0	0%
4.0	24.0	250	na	3.0	na	5	21%
1.0	6.0	60	na	1.0	na	0	26%
2.0	tr	125	na	2.0	na	5	60%
17.0	33.0	770	na	19.0	na	200	46%

Food Name	Serving Size	Total Calories
breakfast sandwich, w/bacon	1 serving	430
breakfast sandwich, w/sausage	1 serving	570
eggs, scrambled	2 eggs	190
French toast	2 slices	400
omelet, ham and cheese	1 serving	290
omelet, ham, cheese, and mushroom ..	1 serving	290
omelet, ham, cheese, onion, and green pepper	1 serving	280
omelet, mushroom, green pepper, and onion	1 serving	210
potatoes	1 serving	360
sausage patty	1 patty	200
BROCCOLI, raw	1/2 cup	12
BUN		
Kaiser	1 bun	180
multigrain	1 bun	140
white	1 bun	140
CABBAGE, red, raw	1/4 cup	4
CANTALOUPE	2 pieces	18
CARROTS, raw	1/4 cup	12
CATSUP	1 tsp	6
CAULIFLOWER, raw	1/2 cup	12
CELERY, raw	1 tbsp	0
CHEESE		
American, salad bar item	1 oz	90
American, sandwich topping	1 slice	60
cheddar, shredded	1 oz	110
imitation, shredded	1 oz	90
mozzarella	1 oz	90
Parmesan, grated	1 oz	130
Parmesan, imitation	1 oz	80
provolone	1 oz	90
Swiss	1 oz	90

Prot. MGS	Carbs. GMS	Sodium MGS	Fiber GMS	Fat GMS	Sat. Fat GMS	Chol. MGS	% Fat Cal.
21.0	33.0	1020	na	23.0	na	na	48%
25.0	33.0	1175	na	37.0	na	na	58%
14.0	7.0	160	na	12.0	na	450	57%
11.0	45.0	850	na	19.0	na	115	43%
18.0	7.0	570	na	21.0	na	355	65%
18.0	7.0	570	na	21.0	na	355	65%
19.0	7.0	485	na	19.0	na	525	61%
14.0	7.0	200	na	15.0	na	460	64%
4.0	37.0	745	na	22.0	na	20	55%
8.0	tr	405	na	18.0	na	45	81%
2.0	2.0	5	na	tr	na	0	0%
7.0	32.0	390	na	2.0	na	5	10%
5.0	25.0	215	na	3.0	na	tr	19%
4.0	26.0	255	na	2.0	na	tr	13%
2.0	tr	5	na	tr	na	0	0%
tr	4.0	5	na	tr	na	0	0%
0.0	2.0	10	na	0.0	0.0	0	0%
tr	1.0	50	na	tr	na	0	0%
1.0	2.0	10	na	tr	na	0	0%
1.0	tr	5	na	tr	na	0	0%
6.0	tr	365	na	7.0	na	5	70%
4.0	tr	295	na	6.0	na	15	90%
7.0	1.0	175	0	10.0	6.0	30	82%
6.0	1.0	125	na	6.0	4.0	0	60%
6.0	tr	335	na	7.0	na	tr	70%
12.0	1.0	510	na	9.0	na	20	62%
9.0	4.0	410	na	3.0	3.0	0	34%
6.0	tr	335	na	7.0	na	tr	70%
6.0	tr	365	na	7.0	na	5	70%

Food Name	Serving Size	Total Calories
CHEESE SAUCE	2 oz	39
CHEESEBURGER		
bacon, 'Jr.' 5.5 oz	1 serving	430
double	1 serving	620
'Jr.' 4.4 oz	1 serving	310
'Jr. Swiss Deluxe' 5.8 oz	1 serving	360
'Kids Meal' 4.1 oz	1 serving	300
CHICKEN NUGGET		
crispy, 6 pieces	1 serving	310
crispy, 9 pieces	1 serving	465
crispy, 20 pieces	1 serving	1023
CHICKEN SANDWICH		
breast, on white bun	1 serving	340
club, 7.2 oz	1 serving	506
fried, 6.9 oz	1 serving	440
grilled, 6.2 oz	1 serving	340
CHILI		
8-oz size	1 serving	190
regular, 9 oz	1 serving	220
12-oz size	1 serving	290
CHIPS		
cheddar	1 oz	160
taco	1.4 oz	260
CHIVES	1/2 tsp	8
CHOW MEIN NOODLES	.5 oz	70
COLESLAW		
'California'	2 tbsp	45
salad bar item	1/4 cup	80
COOKIE, chocolate chip	2.25 oz	275
CORN RELISH, 'Old Fashioned'	1/4 cup	35
COTTAGE CHEESE	1/2 cup	110
CRACKER, saltines, 2 pieces	1 pkt	25
CROUTONS	.5 oz	70

Prot. MGS	Carbs. GMS	Sodium MGS	Fiber GMS	Fat GMS	Sat. Fat GMS	Chol. MGS	% Fat Cal.
1.0	5.0	305	0	2.0	1.0	tr	46%
22.0	33.0	840	(mq)	25.0	5.2	50	52%
48.0	26.0	760	na	36.0	na	165	52%
18.0	34.0	770	(mq)	13.0	3.0	35	38%
18.0	35.0	765	(mq)	18.0	3.0	40	45%
18.0	33.0	770	(mq)	13.0	3.0	35	39%
15.0	14.0	660	na	21.0	na	50	61%
23.0	21.0	990	na	32.0	na	75	62%
50.0	46.0	2178	na	69.0	na	160	61%
26.0	30.0	565	na	12.0	na	60	32%
30.0	43.0	930	(mq)	25.0	4.8	70	44%
26.0	43.0	725	(mq)	19.0	2.6	60	39%
24.0	37.0	815	(mq)	13.0	2.2	60	34%
19.0	21.0	670	na	6.0	na	40	28%
21.0	23.0	750	(mq)	7.0	2.6	45	29%
28.0	31.0	1000	na	9.0	na	60	28%
3.0	12.0	445	na	11.0	na	na	62%
4.0	40.0	20	(mq)	10.0	0.7	0	35%
tr	1.0	na	na	tr	na	0	0%
1.0	8.0	105	na	4.0	na	na	51%
<1.0	5.0	60	na	3.0	<1.0	5	60%
tr	9.0	165	na	5.0	na	40	56%
3.0	40.0	256	(mq)	13.0	4.2	15	43%
tr	9.0	215	na	tr	na	na	0%
13.0	3.0	425	na	4.0	na	20	33%
4.0	1.0	80	na	1.0	na	0	36%
1.0	8.0	105	na	4.0	na	na	51%

Food Name	Serving Size	Total Calories
CUCUMBER	3 slices	2
DANISH		
apple	1 serving	360
cheese	1 serving	430
cinnamon raisin	1 serving	430
EGG, hard-cooked, salad topping	1 tbsp	30
FETTUCCINE	2 oz	190
FISH SANDWICH, fillet, 6 oz	1 serving	460
FRENCH FRIES		
large order	1 serving	390
regular order	1 serving	300
small order, 3.2 oz	1 serving	240
FROZEN DESSERT		
'Frosty Dairy' large	1 serving	680
'Frosty Dairy' small	1 serving	400
GARLIC TOAST	.6-oz piece	70
GRAPEFRUIT	2 oz	10
GRAPES	1/4 cup	30
HAMBURGER		
'Big Classic' on Kaiser bun	1 serving	470
double, 'Big Classic' on Kaiser bun	1 serving	680
double, on white bun	1 serving	560
'Kid's Meal' 3.7 oz	1 serving	260
single, 1/4 lb, on white bun	1 serving	350
single, plain, 4.4 oz	1 serving	340
single, w/everything	1 serving	420
HONEY SAUCE	.5 oz	45
HONEYDEW MELON	2 pieces	20
LETTUCE		
iceberg	1 cup	9
romaine	1 cup	9
sandwich topping	1 leaf	2

Prot. MGS	Carbs. GMS	Sodium MGS	Fiber GMS	Fat GMS	Sat. Fat GMS	Chol. MGS	% Fat Cal.
1.0	tr	na	na	tr	na	0	0%
6.0	53.0	380	na	14.0	na	na	35%
8.0	52.0	550	na	21.0	na	na	44%
8.0	52.0	550	na	21.0	na	na	44%
3.0	tr	25	na	2.0	na	90	60%
4.0	27.0	3	(mq)	3.0	0.6	10	14%
18.0	42.0	780	(mq)	25.0	4.7	50	49%
6.0	46.0	176	na	20.0	na	7	46%
5.0	35.0	135	na	15.0	na	5	45%
3.0	33.0	145	(mq)	12.0	2.5	0	45%
14.0	100.0	374	na	24.0	na	na	32%
8.0	59.0	220	na	14.0	na	50	32%
2.0	9.0	65	(mq)	3.0	0.6	tr	39%
0.0	2.0	0	na	tr	na	0	0%
tr	7.0	na	na	tr	na	0	0%
26.0	36.0	900	na	25.0	na	80	48%
46.0	36.0	1005	na	39.0	na	155	52%
44.0	26.0	465	na	30.0	na	150	48%
15.0	33.0	570	(mq)	9.0	3.0	35	31%
24.0	26.0	360	na	16.0	na	75	41%
24.0	30.0	500	(mq)	15.0	5.5	65	40%
25.0	35.0	890	(mq)	21.0	5.5	70	45%
0.0	12.0	tr	0	0.0	0.0	0	0%
tr	5.0	5	na	tr	na	0	0%
tr	1.0	5	na	tr	na	0	0%
tr	1.0	5	na	tr	na	0	0%
0.0	0.0	tr	na	0.0	na	0	0%

Food Name	Serving Size	Total Calories
MARGARINE		
liquid	.5 oz	100
whipped	1 tbsp	70
MAYONNAISE	1 tbsp	90
MILK, 2%	8 oz	110
MUSHROOMS, raw	1/4 cup	4
MUSTARD	1 tsp	4
MUSTARD SAUCE, sweet	1 oz	50
ONION		
red, raw	3 rings	2
sandwich topping	3 rings	2
ORANGE	2 oz	25
ORANGE JUICE	6 oz	80
PASTA AND NOODLES. See also individual listings.		
medley	2 oz	60
PEACH	2 pieces	17
PEAS, green	1 oz	25
PEPPER, rings	1 tbsp	2
PEPPER, CHERRY, mild	1 tbsp	6
PEPPER, GREEN	1/4 cup	3
PEPPER, JALAPEÑO	1 slice	9
PICANTE SAUCE	2 oz	18
PICKLE, dill	4 slices	2
PINEAPPLE, chunks	1/2 cup	70
POTATO, BAKED		
hot stuffed, w/bacon and cheese	12.8 oz	520
hot stuffed, w/broccoli and cheese	12.3 oz	400
hot stuffed, w/cheese	11.2 oz	420
hot stuffed, w/chili and cheese	14.2 oz	500
hot stuffed, w/sour cream and chives	11.4 oz	500
plain	8.8 oz	270
PUDDING		
butterscotch	1/4 cup	90

Prot. MGS	Carbs. GMS	Sodium MGS	Fiber GMS	Fat GMS	Sat. Fat GMS	Chol. MGS	% Fat Cal.
tr	tr	100	na	11.0	na	0	99%
tr	tr	60	na	8.0	na	0	100%
tr	tr	60	na	10.0	na	10	100%
8.0	11.0	115	na	4.0	na	20	33%
1.0	tr	tr	na	tr	na	0	0%
tr	tr	45	na	tr	na	0	0%
<1.0	9.0	140	(mq)	1.0	<1.0	0	18%
1.0	tr	tr	na	tr	na	0	0%
tr	tr	tr	na	tr	na	0	0%
tr	7.0	0	na	tr	na	0	0%
1.0	19.0	na	na	tr	na	0	0%
2.0	9.0	5	(mq)	2.0	0.3	tr	30%
tr	4.0	0	na	tr	na	0	0%
1.0	4.0	35	na	tr	na	0	0%
tr	tr	200	na	tr	na	0	0%
1.0	tr	180	na	tr	na	0	0%
1.0	1.0	5	na	tr	na	0	0%
tr	2.0	4	na	tr	na	0	0%
<1.0	4.0	5	na	<1.0	<1.0	na	0%
tr	tr	tr	na	tr	na	0	0%
tr	18.0	0	na	tr	na	0	0%
20.0	70.0	1460	(mq)	18.0	5.1	20	31%
8.0	58.0	455	(mq)	16.0	2.9	tr	36%
8.0	66.0	310	(mq)	15.0	4.0	10	32%
15.0	71.0	630	(mq)	18.0	4.0	25	32%
8.0	67.0	135	(mq)	23.0	9.3	25	41%
6.0	63.0	20	(mq)	<1.0	tr	0	0%
1.0	11.0	85	na	4.0	na	tr	40%

Food Name	Serving Size	Total Calories
chocolate	1/4 cup	90
RADISH, raw	.5 oz	2
RAVIOLI, cheese, in sauce	2 oz	45
REFRIED BEANS	2 oz	70
RICE, Spanish	2 oz	70
ROTINI	2 oz	90
SALAD		
Caesar, side order	1 serving	160
chef's	9.1 oz	130
chef's, 'Take Out' approx 11.7 oz	1 serving	180
chicken, grilled	1 serving	200
garden	8.1 oz	70
garden, deluxe	1 serving	110
garden, 'Take Out' approx 9.8 oz	1 serving	102
pasta	1/4 cup	130
pasta, deli	1/4 cup	35
'Pick-Up-Window'	1 serving	110
potato, red bliss	1/4 cup	110
side order	1 serving	60
taco	17.3 oz	530
three bean, deluxe	1/4 cup	60
SALAD DRESSING		
bacon and tomato, reduced calorie	1 tbsp	45
blue cheese, 1 ladle = 2 tbsp	1 tbsp	60
celery seed, 1 ladle = 2 tbsp	1 tbsp	70
creamy cucumber, reduced calorie, 1 ladle = 2 tbsp	1 tbsp	50
French, fat-free, 1/2 pkt = 2 tbsp	2 tbsp	35
French, sweet red	1 tbsp	70
French style, 1 ladle = 2 tbsp	1 tbsp	70
Italian, golden, 1 ladle = 2 tbsp	1 tbsp	50
Italian, reduced calorie	1 tbsp	25
Italian caesar	1 tbsp	80

Prot. MGS	Carbs. GMS	Sodium MGS	Fiber GMS	Fat GMS	Sat. Fat GMS	Chol. MGS	% Fat Cal.
tr	12.0	70	na	4.0	na	tr	40%
1.0	tr	tr	na	tr	na	0	0%
1.0	8.0	290	(mq)	1.0	0.3	5	20%
4.0	10.0	215	(mq)	3.0	0.9	tr	39%
2.0	13.0	440	(mq)	1.0	0.2	tr	13%
3.0	15.0	tr	(mq)	2.0	0.3	tr	20%
10.0	18.0	700	na	6.0	na	10	34%
14.0	8.0	460	(mq)	5.0	1.2	40	35%
15.0	10.0	140	na	9.0	na	120	45%
25.0	9.0	690	na	8.0	na	55	36%
4.0	9.0	60	(mq)	2.0	0.0	0	26%
7.0	9.0	380	na	5.0	na	0	41%
7.0	9.0	110	na	5.0	na	0	44%
3.0	18.0	190	na	6.0	na	5	42%
2.0	6.0	120	na	tr	na	na	0%
8.0	5.0	540	na	6.0	na	0	49%
tr	6.0	265	na	9.0	na	na	74%
4.0	6.0	200	na	3.0	0.0	na	45%
27.0	55.0	825	(mq)	23.0	(mq)	35	39%
1.0	13.0	15	na	tr	na	na	0%
<1.0	3.0	190	na	4.0	0.6	<1	80%
tr	1.0	85	na	6.0	na	10	90%
tr	3.0	65	na	6.0	na	5	77%
tr	2.0	140	na	5.0	na	tr	90%
0.0	8.0	180	na	0.0	na	0	0%
<1.0	5.0	125	na	6.0	0.8	0	77%
tr	5.0	130	na	5.0	na	0	64%
tr	3.0	260	na	4.0	na	0	72%
<1.0	2.0	185	na	2.0	0.3	0	72%
<1.0	<1.0	140	na	8.0	1.4	5	90%

Food Name	Serving Size	Total Calories
oil, 1 ladle = 2 tbsp	1 tbsp	120
ranch, Hidden Valley	1 tbsp	50
Thousand Island, 1 ladle = 2 tbsp	1 tbsp	70
Thousand Island, reduced calorie, 1 ladle = 2 tbsp	1 tbsp	45
wine vinegar, 1 ladle = 2 tbsp	1 tbsp	2
SOUR CREAM		
	1 oz	60
	2 tsp	20
SOUR CREAM, imitation	1 oz	58
SPAGHETTI SAUCE		
regular	1/4 cup	30
w/meat	2 oz	60
STEAK SANDWICH, country-fried, 5.1 oz	1 serving	440
STRAWBERRIES	2 oz	18
SUNFLOWER SEEDS, w/raisins	1 oz	140
SWEET AND SOUR SAUCE	1 oz	45
SYRUP	1 pkt	140
TACO MEAT	2 oz	110
TACO SAUCE	1 oz	16
TACO SHELL	.4 oz	45
TARTAR SAUCE	1 tbsp	80
TOMATO, 1-oz slice	1 slice	6
TORTELLINI, cheese, in sauce	2 oz	60
TORTILLA, flour 1.3 oz	1 tortilla	110
TURKEY HAM	1/4 cup	50
WATERMELON	3 pieces	18

WHATABURGER

APPLE PIE	1 serving	236
APPLE TURNOVER	1 serving	215
BISCUIT, buttermilk	1 serving	280

Prot. MGS	Carbs. GMS	Sodium MGS	Fiber GMS	Fat GMS	Sat. Fat GMS	Chol. MGS	% Fat Cal.
tr	tr	0	na	14.0	na	0	100%
<1.0	<1.0	95	na	5.0	1.0	5	90%
tr	tr	115	na	7.0	na	10	90%
tr	2.0	125	na	4.0	na	5	80%
tr	tr	5	na	tr	na	0	0%
1.0	1.0	15	0	6.0	3.6	10	90%
tr	tr	5	na	2.0	na	5	90%
<1.0	2.0	30	0	5.0	5.0	0	78%
1.0	6.0	340	na	<1.0	<1.0	0	0%
4.0	8.0	315	(mq)	2.0	0.7	10	30%
14.0	45.0	870	(mq)	25.0	5.7	35	51%
tr	4.0	tr	na	tr	na	0	0%
5.0	6.0	5	na	10.0	na	0	64%
<1.0	11.0	55	na	<1.0	tr	0	0%
tr	37.0	5	na	tr	na	0	0%
10.0	4.0	300	na	7.0	1.7	25	57%
<1.0	3.0	140	na	<1.0	tr	tr	0%
<1.0	6.0	45	(mq)	3.0	0.7	0	60%
tr	tr	75	na	9.0	na	na	100%
1.0	1.0	5	na	tr	na	0	0%
2.0	12.0	280	(mq)	1.0	0.3	5	15%
3.0	19.0	220	(mq)	3.0	0.4	na	25%
6.0	tr	na	na	2.0	na	na	36%
tr	4.0	tr	na	tr	na	0	0%
3.0	30.0	265	na	12.0	na	tr	46%
2.4	27.0	241	na	10.8	na	0	45%
5.4	36.6	509	na	13.4	na	3	43%

Food Name	Serving Size	Total Calories
BREAKFAST		
bacon	1 slice	38
biscuit, w/bacon	1 serving	359
biscuit, w/egg and cheese	1 serving	434
biscuit, w/egg, cheese, and bacon	1 serving	511
biscuit, w/egg, cheese, and sausage	1 serving	601
biscuit, w/gravy	1 serving	479
biscuit, w/sausage	1 serving	446
eggs, scrambled	2 eggs	189
pancakes	3 pancakes	259
pancakes, w/sausage	3 pancakes	426
pancakes, w/o syrup or butter	1 serving	259
platter, w/bacon	1 serving	695
platter, w/sausage	1 serving	785
sausage	1 serving	208
BREAKFAST SANDWICH		
'Breakfast on a Bun'	1 serving	520
'Breakfast on a Bun' ranchero	1 serving	530
'Breakfast on a Bun' w/bacon	1 serving	365
egg omelette	1 serving	288
egg omelette 'Ranchero'	1 serving	322
BUN		
5-inch size	1 bun	290
4-inch size	1 bun	150
BUTTER	1 pkt	36
CHEESEBURGER		
double meat	1 serving	895
'Jr. Burger'	1 serving	351
'Justaburger'	1 serving	312
regular	1 serving	669
CHICKEN SANDWICH		
grilled	1 serving	442
grilled, w/o salad dressing	1 serving	385

Prot. MGS	Carbs. GMS	Sodium MGS	Fiber GMS	Fat GMS	Sat. Fat GMS	Chol. MGS	% Fat Cal.
2.0	0.0	106	na	3.3	na	6	78%
9.6	36.7	730	na	20.2	na	15	51%
13.7	37.5	797	na	26.3	na	202	55%
17.8	37.6	1010	na	32.9	na	213	58%
20.7	37.9	1081	na	41.6	na	236	62%
8.8	48.3	1253	na	27.4	na	20	51%
12.3	37.0	794	na	28.7	na	37	58%
11.3	1.5	211	na	15.0	na	374	71%
10.6	39.9	842	na	5.8	na	0	20%
17.5	40.3	1127	na	21.1	na	34	45%
11.0	40.0	842	na	6.0	na	0	21%
22.1	54.1	1162	na	44.0	na	389	57%
24.9	54.4	1234	na	52.7	na	412	60%
9.0	1.0	355	na	19.0	na	43	82%
23.0	29.0	1051	na	34.0	na	234	59%
23.0	32.0	1431	na	35.0	na	236	59%
17.5	29.4	815	na	19.4	na	210	48%
13.4	29.4	602	na	12.8	na	198	40%
15.0	31.0	1067	na	16.0	na	191	45%
10.0	56.0	532	na	3.0	na	tr	9%
5.0	29.0	274	na	2.0	na	tr	12%
0.0	0.0	42	na	4.0	na	11	100%
55.0	59.0	1678	na	49.0	na	180	49%
17.0	30.0	921	na	18.0	na	42	46%
15.0	28.0	784	na	16.0	na	37	46%
36.0	58.0	1474	na	33.0	na	96	44%
34.3	48.4	1103	na	14.2	na	66	29%
34.0	46.0	989	na	9.0	na	66	21%

Food Name	Serving Size	Total Calories
'Whatachick'n Deluxe'	1 serving	573
COFFEE, small	1 serving	5
COOKIE		
chocolate chunk	1 cookie	247
macadamia nut	1 cookie	269
oatmeal raisin	1 cookie	222
peanut butter	1 cookie	262
CRACKER, Club	1 pkt	31
CREAMER, nondairy	1 pkg	10
CROUTONS	1 pkt	29
FAJITA TACO		
beef	1 serving	326
chicken	1 serving	272
FISH SANDWICH		
'Whatacatch'	1 serving	475
'Whatacatch' w/cheese	1 serving	522
FRENCH FRIES		
junior order	1 serving	221
large order	1 serving	442
regular order	1 serving	332
HAMBURGER		
'Justaburger'	1 serving	265
'Whataburger'	1 serving	598
'Whataburger' w/double meat	1 serving	823
HAMBURGER PATTY		
ground beef, 1/4 lb	1 patty	226
ground beef, 1/10 lb	1 patty	90
HONEY	1 pkt	27
ICED TEA, med	1 serving	3
JAM, strawberry	1 pkt	37
JELLY, grape	1 pkt	38
LEMON JUICE	1 pkt	1
MARGARINE	1 pkt	25

Prot. MGS	Carbs. GMS	Sodium MGS	Fiber GMS	Fat GMS	Sat. Fat GMS	Chol. MGS	% Fat Cal.
34.2	53.0	1338	na	26.9	na	56	42%
0.2	0.9	5	na	0.0	na	0	0%
4.0	28.0	75	na	16.0	na	36	58%
3.0	31.0	80	na	16.0	na	34	54%
4.0	36.9	70	na	7.0	na	28	28%
5.4	30.2	35	na	13.5	na	39	46%
0.5	3.9	72	na	1.3	na	0	38%
0.0	1.0	4	na	1.0	na	0	90%
0.9	4.5	88	na	0.9	na	0	28%
21.6	33.6	670	na	11.9	na	28	33%
18.2	35.2	691	na	6.7	na	33	22%
14.0	43.0	722	na	27.0	na	34	51%
16.0	43.0	959	na	32.0	na	45	55%
4.0	25.0	50	na	12.0	na	(tr)	49%
7.1	49.2	292	na	24.2	na	0	49%
5.0	37.0	45	na	18.0	na	(tr)	49%
12.0	28.0	547	na	12.0	na	25	41%
30.2	61.1	1096	na	26.0	na	84	39%
48.9	61.8	1298	na	42.4	na	168	46%
19.0	1.0	232	na	17.0	na	84	68%
8.0	tr	81	na	6.0	na	34	60%
0.0	7.0	0	na	0.0	na	0	0%
0.0	1.0	10	na	0.0	na	0	0%
0.0	9.0	0	na	0.0	na	0	0%
0.0	9.0	0	na	0.0	na	0	0%
0.0	0.3	1	na	0.0	na	0	0%
0.0	0.0	40	na	3.0	na	0	100%

Food Name	Serving Size	Total Calories
MILK, 2% butterfat	1 serving	113
MILKSHAKE		
chocolate, small	1 serving	333
strawberry, small	1 serving	322
vanilla, extra large	1 serving	877
vanilla, large	1 serving	657
vanilla, medium	1 serving	439
vanilla, small	1 serving	322
MUFFIN, blueberry	1 muffin	239
ONION RINGS		
large order	1 serving	493
regular order	1 serving	226
ORANGE JUICE	6 oz	77
PECAN DANISH	1 serving	270
PEPPER, JALAPEÑO	1 pepper	3
PICANTE SAUCE	1 pkt	5
POTATO, BAKED		
plain	1 serving	310
w/broccoli cheese topping	1 serving	453
w/cheese topping	1 serving	510
w/mushroom topping	1 serving	360
POTATOES, HASH BROWN	1 serving	150
SALAD		
chicken, grilled	1 serving	150
garden	1 serving	56
SALAD DRESSING		
French	1 pkt	249
ranch	1 pkt	364
Thousand Island	1 pkt	280
vinaigrette, lite, 2 oz	1 pkt	36
SOFT DRINK		
Cherry Coke, medium size	1 serving	151
Coca-Cola Classic, medium size	1 serving	141

Prot. MGS	Carbs. GMS	Sodium MGS	Fiber GMS	Fat GMS	Sat. Fat GMS	Chol. MGS	% Fat Cal.
8.0	11.0	113	na	4.0	na	18	32%
8.3	56.2	155	na	8.4	na	32	23%
7.8	54.9	152	na	8.0	na	31	22%
25.0	137.0	1168	na	26.0	na	100	27%
19.0	102.0	874	na	19.0	na	75	26%
12.0	68.0	230	na	13.0	na	51	27%
9.0	50.0	169	na	9.0	na	37	25%
6.2	35.6	538	na	7.9	na	0	30%
8.0	50.7	893	na	28.7	na	0	52%
4.0	22.0	410	na	13.0	na	(tr)	52%
1.0	18.0	2	na	0.0	na	0	0%
5.0	28.0	419	na	16.0	na	12	53%
0.1	0.6	190	na	0.1	na	0	30%
0.2	0.9	130	na	0.0	na	0	0%
6.5	71.7	23	na	0.3	na	0	1%
12.9	79.3	636	na	10.0	na	17	20%
14.6	79.8	863	na	16.3	na	22	29%
8.0	80.0	778	na	1.6	na	0	4%
1.3	15.9	228	na	9.0	na	0	54%
23.0	14.0	434	na	1 0	na	49	6%
2.9	11.3	32	na	0.6	na	0	10%
0.0	16.0	729	na	20.0	na	5	72%
0.0	4.0	599	na	37.9	na	5	94%
0.0	9.0	399	na	26.9	na	0	86%
0.0	5.0	878	na	2.0	na	0	50%
0.0	39.6	7	na	0.0	na	0	0%
0.0	37.6	13	na	0.0	na	0	0%

Food Name	Serving Size	Total Calories
Diet Coke, medium size	1 serving	1
Dr. Pepper, medium size	1 serving	138
root beer, medium size	1 serving	158
Sprite, medium size	1 serving	141
SOUR CREAM	2 oz	121
STEAK SANDWICH	1 serving	387
SUGAR	1 pkt	15
SUGAR SUBSTITUTE, 'Sweet 'n Low'	1 pkt	4
SYRUP, pancake	1 pkt	169
TAQUITO		
bacon	1 serving	335
potato	1 serving	446
'Ranchero'	1 serving	320
regular	1 serving	310
sausage	1 serving	443
w/cheese	1 serving	357
w/cheese 'Ranchero'	1 serving	367
TURKEY SANDWICH, grilled	1 serving	439

WHITE CASTLE

Food Name	Serving Size	Total Calories
BREAKFAST SANDWICH		
sausage, 1.7 oz	1 serving	196
sausage and egg, 3.4 oz	1 serving	322
BUN, hamburger, .9 oz	1 bun	74
CHEESE	.3 oz	31
CHEESEBURGER, 2.3 oz	1 serving	200
CHICKEN SANDWICH, 2.3 oz	1 serving	186
CHIPS, 3.3 oz	1 serving	329
FISH SANDWICH, w/o tartar sauce, 2.1 oz	1 serving	155
FRENCH FRIES, 3.4 oz	1 serving	301

Prot. MGS	Carbs. GMS	Sodium MGS	Fiber GMS	Fat GMS	Sat. Fat GMS	Chol. MGS	% Fat Cal.
0.0	0.3	17	na	0.0	na	0	0%
0.0	34.9	34	na	0.3	na	0	2%
0.0	41.7	17	na	0.0	na	0	0%
0.0	31.6	30	na	0.0	na	0	0%
1.8	2.4	30	na	11.9	na	25	89%
35.0	32.0	1164	na	12.0	na	61	28%
0.0	4.0	0	na	0.0	na	0	0%
0.0	1.0	0	na	0.0	na	0	0%
0.0	41.8	0	na	0.0	na	0	0%
14.9	31.7	761	na	16.1	na	286	43%
14.2	47.6	883	na	21.8	na	281	44%
19.0	19.0	1092	na	18.0	na	223	51%
19.0	17.0	712	na	19.0	na	223	55%
19.8	32.1	790	na	25.9	na	315	53%
21.0	17.0	949	na	23.0	na	235	58%
21.0	19.0	1329	na	23.0	na	235	56%
33.0	49.0	968	na	15.0	na	46	31%
7.0	13.0	488	2.0	12.0	(mq)	(mq)	55%
13.0	16.0	698	3.0	22.0	(mq)	(mq)	61%
2.2	13.9	<1	.5	0.9	na	0	11%
1.5	2.3	154	.2	1.6	(mq)	na	46%
8.0	15.0	361	2.7	11.0	(mq)	(mq)	50%
8.0	21.0	497	1.7	7.0	(mq)	(mq)	34%
4.0	39.0	832	3.5	17.0	(mq)	na	47%
6.0	21.0	201	1.4	5.0	(mq)	(mq)	29%
2.0	38.0	193	4.6	15.0	(mq)	na	45%

Food Name	Serving Size	Total Calories
HAMBURGER, 2.0 oz	1 serving	161
ONION RINGS, 2.1 oz	1 serving	245

ZANTIGO

BURRITO
hot cheese, 'Chilito'	1 serving	329
mild cheese, 'Chilito'	1 serving	330

ENCHILADA
beef	1 serving	315
cheese	1 serving	390

TACO
burrito	1 serving	415
regular	1 serving	198

Prot. MGS	Carbs. GMS	Sodium MGS	Fiber GMS	Fat GMS	Sat. Fat GMS	Chol. MGS	% Fat Cal.
6.0	15.0	266	2.1	8.0	(mq)	(mq)	45%
3.0	27.0	566	2.6	13.0	(mq)	na	48%
14.0	35.0	466	na	15.0	na	na	41%
14.0	36.0	505	na	15.0	na	na	41%
18.0	26.0	904	na	15.0	na	na	43%
20.0	26.0	759	na	23.0	na	na	53%
21.0	41.0	815	na	19.0	na	na	41%
10.0	13.0	318	na	12.0	na	na	55%

NUTRiBASE Software for PC's

NutriBase for Windows provides you with the world's largest database of food items, then helps you set and track your nutritional goals. Goals that help you achieve not only your ideal body weight, but a diet that conforms with national dietary guidelines (or any other guidelines).

NutriBase provides lightning-fast access to nutritional information for 47,547 foods. The Personal Version tracks *calories, protein, carbohydrates, total fat, % calories from fat, saturated fat, sodium, cholesterol, fiber,* and *alcohol.* NutriBase Professional tracks all of these plus 85 additional nutrients. The following capabilities are your keys to a healthier lifestyle:

 Users - NutriBase tracks the progress for up to 5 users (200 in the Pro version). Answer a few questions and NutriBase suggests nutrition and body weight goals. Then NutriBase helps you track the data for everything you eat.

 View - Click on this icon to display alphabetized views of *17,000 generic and 31,000 brand named foods,* including *3,160 menu items from over 70 restaurants.*

 Rank - Instantly rank foods based on their values for any nutrient. For instance, rank the 500 or so breakfast cereals from high-to-low based on their fiber content.

 Query - Instantly locate *all* foods that meet *all* the criteria that *you* specify. The NutriBase query function is more flexible and powerful than *any* similar capability of *any* competing nutrition package at *any* price... Guaranteed.

 Frequent Food Item - Use this icon to create an alphabetical list of your most commonly eaten foods. NutriBase also allows you to add new food items.

 Recipes - Drag and drop ingredients into this icon to create recipes. Edit ingredients, specify serving sizes, view nutrient data, graph it, print it, save it, and more.